Tendon transfer for irreparable cuff tear

Springer

Paris
Berlin
Heidelberg
New York
Hong Kong
Londres
Milan
Tokyo

Philippe Valenti

Tendon transfer for irreparable cuff tear

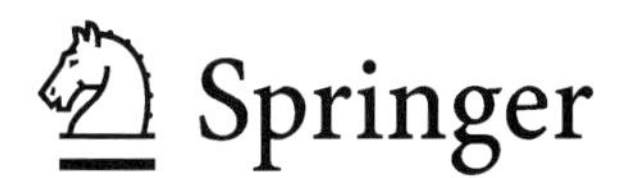

Philippe Valenti
Orthopaedic Surgery – Shoulder, elbow and hand
Institut de la Main
6, square Jouvenet
75016 Paris
France

ISBN : 978-2-8178-0048-6 Springer Paris Berlin Heidelberg New York

Springer-Verlag France est membre du groupe Springer Science + Business Media

Cover design: Nadia Ouddane
Cover Illustration: Anne Saunier
Lay-out: Desk

"GECO" book series coordinated by P. Kehr

The aim of the "GECO" book series, to which this book belongs, is to perpetuate the work of GECO "Groupe d'études pour la Chirurgie osseuse" (Group for the Study of Bone surgery) and to celebrate the thirty years of existence of the group.

Born in 1976, GECO was at the beginning the meeting place of a group of young surgeons in orthopedics and traumatology who brought together their patient files in order to carry out prospective studies and improve their knowledge.

Very soon the group, through an annual meeting that was organized with the support of Fournitures Hospitaliers (FH Orthopedics), gathered in January of each year a growing number of orthopedic surgeons from Europe - over 300 at present - at its round tables and its oral presentations, mostly from France but also from all over the world.

GECO today is a group of over 25 permanent members and six specialty groups representing the major sub-specialties of orthopedics and traumatology. With a regular publication rhythm of one to two books per year, the GECO has given himself given as a goal to provide the community of orthopedic surgery the fruit of his reflections and its work.

In the same book series:

Dambreville A., Dubrana F., Kehr P., Petit R. *et al.*, *Les prothèses de hanche sans ciment de première intention. Techniques opératoires. Problèmes et solutions.* Springer-Verlag France, Paris 2004.

Gacon G., Humer J., *Les prothèses tricompartimentaires du genou de première intention. Techniques opératoires. Problèmes et solutions.* Springer-Verlag France, Paris 2006.

Favreul E., Dambreville A., Gacon G., Kehr P., *Classifications et scores en chirurgie orthopédique et en traumatologie. Volume 1 : rachis, hanche, cuisse, genou.* Springer-Verlag France, Paris 2008.

Thanks to:

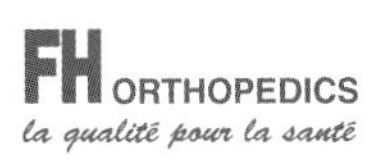

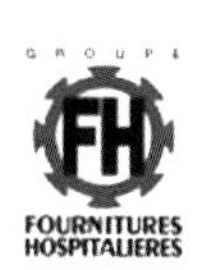

(www.f-h.fr)

for its contribution and its financial support.

The illustrations in the following chapters have been drawn by Marc Donon.

Chapters:
- *Results of latissimus dorsi tendon in primary…*
- *Arthroscopic humeral head interference screw fixation…*
- *Deltoid flap for irreparable rotator cuff tear…*
- *The myotendinous advancements of supra and infraspinatus muscles…*
- *Transfer of the pectoralis major…*
- *Reverse shoulder prosthesis combined with latissimus dorsi…*

Illustrations: Marc Donon – Illustration médicale
mdonon@mac.com

Contributors

Yves Bellumore
Department of Orthopaedics and Traumatology
Clinique d'Occitanie
20, avenue Bernard IV
31605 Muret
France

Eric Berthonnaud
Engineer – Shoulder and Elbow Unit
Herriot Hospital
5, Place d'Arsonval
69437 Lyon Cedex 03
France

Luis-Carlos Diaz
Institut de la Main
6, square Jouvenet
75016 Paris
France

Michel Colmar
Centre Hospitalier Privé de Saint-Brieuc
Clinique Sainte Jeanne d'Arc
9, rue du Vieux Séminaire
22000 Saint-Brieuc
France

Joannès Dimnet
Engineer – Shoulder and Elbow Unit
Herriot Hospital
5, Place d'Arsonval
69437 Lyon Cedex 03
France

A. Dotziz
Department of Orthopaedics and Traumatology
CHU Dupuytren
2, avenue Martin Luther King
87042 Limoges Cedex
France

Sebastian Ferriere
Department of Orthopaedics and Traumatology
University Hospital Centre of Toulouse-Purpan
Place du Docteur Baylac
31059 Toulouse
France

Jérôme Garret
Orthopaedic surgery – Shoulder, elbow and hand
Clinique du Parc
155, boulevard Stalingrad
69006 Lyon
France

Jean-Emmanuel Gedouin
Nouvelles cliniques Nantaises
3, rue Eric Tabarly
44277 Nantes Cedex
France

Sophie Grosclaude
Orthopaedic surgery – Shoulder, elbow and hand
Clinique du Parc
155, boulevard Stalingrad
69006 Lyon
France

Guillaume Herzberg
Head of Shoulder and Elbow Unit
Herriot Hospital
5, Place d'Arsonval
69437 Lyon Cedex 03
France

Ibrahim Kalouche
Department of Orthopaedic Surgery
CHU Bicêtre
78, rue du Général Leclerc
94270 Le Kremlin-Bicêtre
France

Jean Kany
Department of Orthopaedic and
Traumatological Surgery
Nouvelle clinique de l'union
Boulevard de Ratalens
31240 Saint-Jean
France

Alim Kaouar
Clinique Jouvenet
Institut de la Main
6, square Jouvenet
75016 Paris
France

Denis Katz
Department of Orthopaedic and
Traumatological Surgery
Clinique du Ter
BP 71
56275 Plœmeur Cedex
France

Alexandre Kilinc
Department of Orthopaedic Surgery
Saint-Antoine Hospital
184, rue du Faubourg Saint-Antoine
75012 Paris
France

H.-A. Kumar
Department of Orthopaedic and
Traumatological Surgery
Nouvelle clinique de l'union
Boulevard de Ratalens
31240 Saint-Jean
France

Christophe Lévigne
Shoulder Department
Clinique du Parc
155, boulevard Stalingrad
69006 Lyon
France

Michel Mansat
Department of Orthopaedics and
Traumatology
University Hospital Centre
of Toulouse-Purpan
Place du Docteur Baylac
31059 Toulouse
France

Pierre Mansat
Department of Orthopaedics and
Traumatology
University Hospital Centre
of Toulouse-Purpan
Place du Docteur Baylac
31059 Toulouse
France

Jean-Marie Postel
Department of Orthopaedic and
Traumatological Surgery
Clinique Arago
96, boulevard Arago
75014 Paris
France

Philippe Sauzières
Institut de la Main
6, square Jouvenet
75016 Paris
France

Oliver Schoierer
Shoulder and Elbow Unit
Herriot Hospital
5, Place d'Arsonval
69437 Lyon Cedex 03
France

Hervé Thomazeau
General Surgery
CHRU Hôpital Sud
16, boulevard de Bulgarie
BP 90347
35203 Rennes Cedex 2
France

Laurent Thomsen
Department of Orthopaedic and
Traumatological Surgery
Saint-Antoine Hospital
184, rue Faubourg Saint-Antoine
75012 Paris
France

Jean-Pierre Urien
Shoulder and Elbow Unit
Herriot Hospital
5, Place d'Arsonval
69437 Lyon Cedex 03
France

Philippe Valenti
Orthopaedic surgery – Shoulder, elbow and hand
Institut de la Main
6, square Jouvenet
75016 Paris
France

Contents

Foreword

In the last twenty-five years the diagnosis and treatment of rotator cuff tears have seen tremendous progress. Whereas in the 1960ies surgeons believed that all ruptures are reparable and are amenable to a successful outcome, experience and conscientious follow-up studies have taught us differently: Many rotator cuff repairs fail to heal and indeed the majority of large rotator cuff tears do either not or only partially heal.

Imaging has changed rotator cuff tear management: It has allowed for classification of the extent of tendon tear and quantification of associated changes, namely the degree of muscular changes caused by tendon tearing. Computed tomography, magnetic resonance imaging with and without arthrography and ultrasound have allowed a relatively reliable prediction of healing of a given rotator cuff tear. The imaging modalities have also allowed an in depth study of the outcome of as well the tendon repairs as of the muscular (non-) recovery of the affected motors of the shoulder joint.

What has been established?

- It has been established that *irreparable rotator cuff tears do exist*. There are defects which even the most dexterous orthopaedic surgeon can not close intraoperatively and tears which consistently fail to heal despite successful intraoperative repair.
- It has been established that *irreparable rotator cuff tears can preoperatively be identified*. Tears which are associated with chronic cranial migration of the humeral head or so – called "static glenohumeral subluxation" and advanced fatty infiltration of the rotator cuff muscles will not heal, even if defect closure was possible intraoperatively. These tears must be considered irreparable.
- *Some irreparable tears are best left untreated*. Many patients with irreparable tears suffer relatively little, live up to their functional demands without substantial suffering and in fact may be made worse by attempts at cuff repair.

– *Some irreparable tears cause severe, painful disability and the patients desire treatment.* For pseudoparalysis of anterior elevation in the elderly, the reverse prostheses appear established and uncontested.

What does this book establish?

This book recognizes that there is a surprisingly large population of patients which is sufficiently disabled to warrant treatment for irreparable rotator cuff lesions and for which neither neglect, nor debridement nor reverse prostheses are adequate. There are patients who need pain relief and restoration of as much function as possible and for which the use of tendon transfers is currently the only alternative.

It is not a coincidence that this book is edited and largely written by a hand surgeon and contains multiple authors who have profound knowledge in hand surgery. Tendon transfers have been widely used in functional restoration of the hand. Hand surgeons do not only have the basic understanding of the biomechanics and biology of musculo-tendinous transfer but also the experience of the enormous potential and success of this concept.

This book is both necessary and timely. It adds an extremely valuable element to the shoulder literature and should be carefully studied by all orthopaedic surgeons treating irreparable rotator cuff tears. Although I personally have been working for many years on this subject I would like to thank the editor and the authors, I have learnt a lot reading your chapters.

Christian Gerber, MD, FRCS
Chairman, Dept of orthopaedics, University of Zürich, Switzerland

Biomechanical analysis of tendon transfers for irreparable rotator cuff tears

G. Herzberg, O. Schoierer, E. Berthonnaud, J. Dimnet, J.-P. Urien

Introduction

Musculo-tendinous transfers (MTTs) to treat massive irreparable rotator cuff tears have been proposed since the eighties (1) and are still the subject of considerable interest in the recent literature (2-29). A musculo-tendinous transfer is that procedure in which the tendon of insertion of a normal "donor" muscle with blood and nerve supply intact is divided and reinserted into a bony part or into another tendon (with or without intercalated tendon graft) to supplement or substitute for the action of a non-functioning "recipient" muscle. Before their use in the treatment of irreparable rotator cuff tears, MTT were routinely used to treat muscle palsies. When dealing with irreparable rotator cuff tears, the idea is to provide a new structurally normal muscle with proper vector and torque for restoring the lost function. The application of several fundamental biomechanical principles is essential for a successful MTT (30). Corrections of joint contracture, expandable donor, good local tissues, no tension on the neurovascular pedicle in any position, and one tendon-one function are well-known principles. In addition to these principles, the MTT must be sufficiently strong and have enough amplitude of tendon excursion to perform its new function in its altered position. This means that biomechanical properties (architecture and power) of transferred muscle(s) should be adequate. Ideally potential excursion and power of MTT should match those of the non-functioning recipient muscle(s). Because muscles in general are highly specialized for their function (31) it is almost impossible to find within the shoulder muscles an expandable unit that exactly matches a non-functioning one. There is a relationship between potential excursion and power of any striated muscle (30) (Fig. 1). The maximum tension a muscle fiber can produce is at its resting length, i.e., close to the middle of its potential excursion (Fig. 1). Excursion of a transferred muscle may adapt to its new function with time (32). Knowledge of structural properties of muscle(s) to be replaced and to be transferred may be useful in clinical practice when planning MTT to treat irreparable rotator cuff tears (33). Lastly, the MTT should have a straight line of pull that implies that the choice of its point of transferred fixation is critical (34).

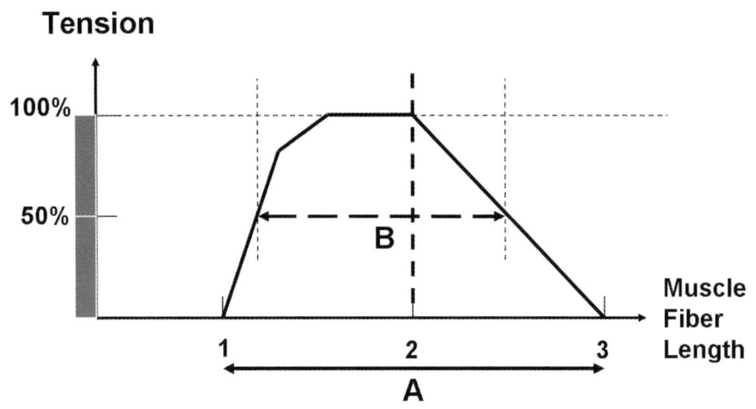

Fig. 1 – Blix curve, or general shape of active contraction of a muscle fiber (modified from Brand PW, *Clinical Mechanics of the Hand*, 1993): a muscle can produce its greatest tension at its resting length, and the force it can produce decreases when it gets shorter or longer. (A) Muscle excursion or resting length and (B) portion of excursion where the muscle can produce between 50 and 100% of its force, (1) muscle length in maximum contraction, (2) muscle length at rest, and (3) muscle length maximally stretched.

The purpose of this study was twofold: first to provide a list of shoulder muscle capabilities in terms of potential excursion (muscle fibers resting length, i.e., muscle excursion without reference to connective tissue restraints) and relative tension (of physiologic cross-sectional areas (PCSAs) expressed in percentage among a group of muscles) that could assist the decision making when planning MTT (33). The second purpose was to discuss the best point of distal fixation of one of the most popular MTTs used to treat irreparable cuff tears, i.e., the latissimus dorsi transfer (34).

Material and methods

Study of biomechanical properties of shoulder girdle muscles

Thirteen shoulder girdle muscles were dissected in 13 fresh cadavers (6 females and 7 males) with intact rotator cuff (33). Ages ranged from 17 to 89 (mean = 74). Four of the 13 muscles (trapezius, serratus anterior, deltoid, and pectoralis major) were divided into bellies because some of these bellies may be used individually as MTT. We will consider only the muscles that are relevant to rotator cuff surgery. The deltoid muscle was divided into four parts: the anterior deltoid arising from the lateral third of the clavicle, the middle deltoid (anterior part) arising from the anterior border of the acromion, the middle deltoid (posterior part) arising from the lateral border of the acromion, and the posterior deltoid arising from the spine of the scapula. The pectoralis major was divided into two parts: the clavicular portion arised from the medial third of the clavicle, whereas the sternocostal portion arised from the entire length of the manubrium, from the aponeurosis of the external oblique muscle, and from the cartilages of the first six ribs. Brand et al.'s method (32) was used to study in each muscle (or muscle belly) the potential excursion (average muscle fiber length measured with 4.3 optical magnification and expressed in centimeters) and relative tension (PCSA of each muscle expressed as a percentage within the group). In longitudinally arranged muscles, fiber length was measured at the two borders and in the middle of the muscle. In pennate and multipennate muscles, the tendon was first traced back into its muscle. Two clamps were attached to both sides of the tendon from its proximal tip to its point of exit from the muscle. The tendon was then cut longitudinally allowing the pennate muscle fibers to be measured from their origin to their insertion to the tendon. In multipennate muscles, measurements were made on each pennated unit and then averaged. To get a realistic PCSA, it was very important to measure the muscle fiber length taking into account the pennation rather than measuring the whole length of the muscle. The fleshy part of each muscle was then weighed. For a given muscle, the percentage of the total weight of the 13 muscles was the mass fraction. The mass of each muscle was converted to volume according to a 1.02 muscle density (32), then divided by the mean fiber length to get the PCSA. In each cadaver, the PCSA were expressed as percentages providing relative tensions figures.

Study of the point of fixation of latissimus dorsi MTT

A right scapula and humerus were harvested from a fresh cadaver and mounted together in a frame, simulating the position of these two bones in the "zero" clinical position of the shoulder (Fig. 2). Steel balls were inserted at the center of the humeral head footprint areas of the supraspinatus, infraspinatus, and teres minor as defined by recent works (35) (Fig. 2). The center areas of origin of the infraspinatus muscle in the infrascapular fossa and of the latissimus dorsi close to the inferior tip of the scapula were also modelized with steel markers. The geometric center of the humeral head was considered as the center of rotation of the simulated joint so that the generated torque could be calculated. Stereoradiography (36) was used to obtain from two standard

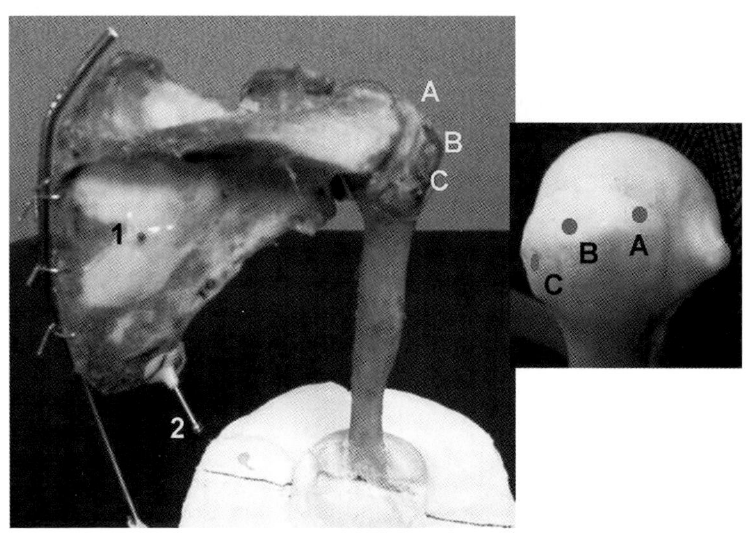

Fig. 2 – Scapula-humerus construct with imbedded steel balls are used to define muscles vectors for modelization (1: origin of infraspinatus vector, 2: origin of latissimus dorsi vector, A: modelized supraspinatus footprint, B: modelized infraspinatus footprint, and C: modelized teres minor footprint).

radiographs (Fig. 3) a three-dimensional modelization of the muscle vectors of innate infraspinatus and latissimus dorsi transfer with fixation on either supraspinatus, infraspinatus, or teres minor footprints. A comparison of vectors in the four situations with the humerus in three positions (neutral, 60° internal rotation, and 50° external rotation) was possible (34). Each muscle vector was studied in three series of 0-90° modelized abduction in the scapular plane. In each series, abduction/adduction and external/internal rotation moment arms were calculated by increments of 3°. "Rolling up" of the force vectors around the humeral head was taken into account. Theoretical muscle forces obtained from the first part of the study were used for muscle torque calculations. The

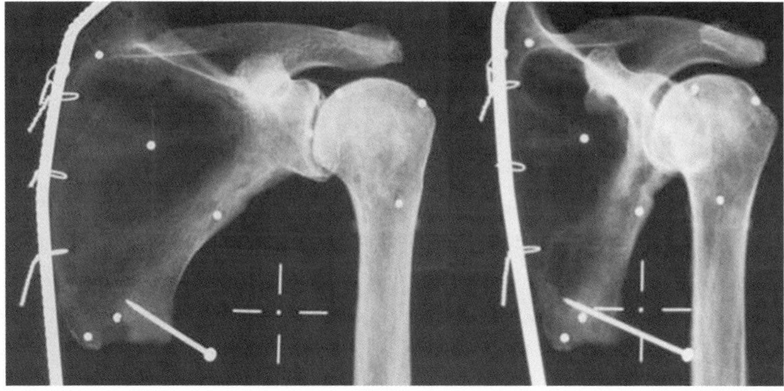

Fig. 3 – Stereoradiographic technique requires one antero-posterior and one oblique views. Extra steel balls are used to modelize bones.

figure used for muscle force-producing capability was 3.6 kg for 1 cm^2 of PCSA of muscle (32). In addition, a video of a latissimus dorsi MTT in a fresh cadaver with fixation on either supraspinatus or infraspinatus humeral head insertions and 0-90° abduction motion in 50° external rotation or 60° internal rotation was performed.

Results

Comparative biomechanical properties of shoulder girdle muscles

Our findings about potential excursion (cm) and relative tension (%) of deltoid, rotator cuff muscles and potential MTT are shown in Figs. 4 and 5. Relative tension is expressed in percentage among the whole group of 13 shoulder girdle muscles. Among rotator cuff muscles, the subscapularis had the greatest relative tension (14.5%). It was well balanced by the combination of infraspinatus and teres minor relative tensions (12.3%). Generally speaking, it should be noted that rotator cuff muscles were short excursion and high relative tension muscles whereas potential MTT demonstrated larger excursions but limited relative tensions (33).

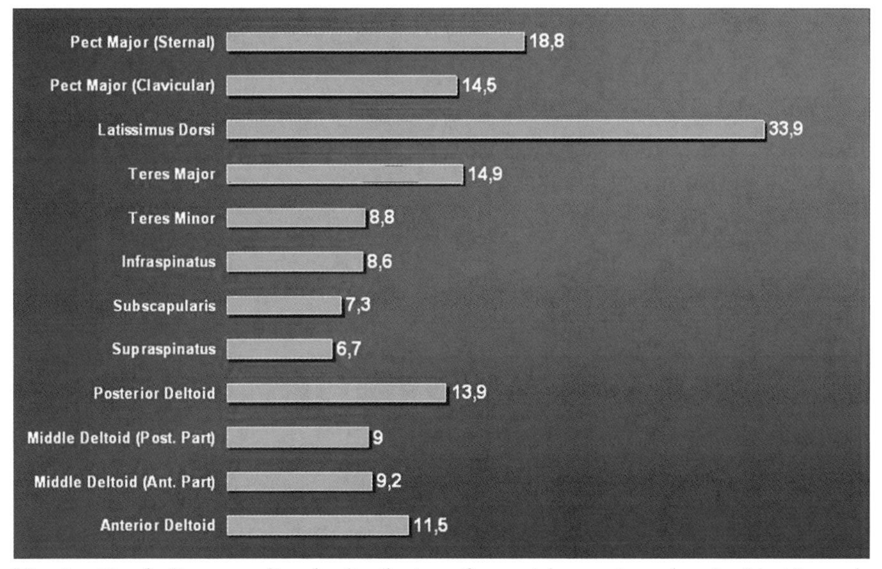

Fig. 4 – Our findings regarding the distribution of potential excursion values (cm) in 12 muscle bellies of the shoulder girdle that may be involved in tendon transfers, either as recipients or as donors.

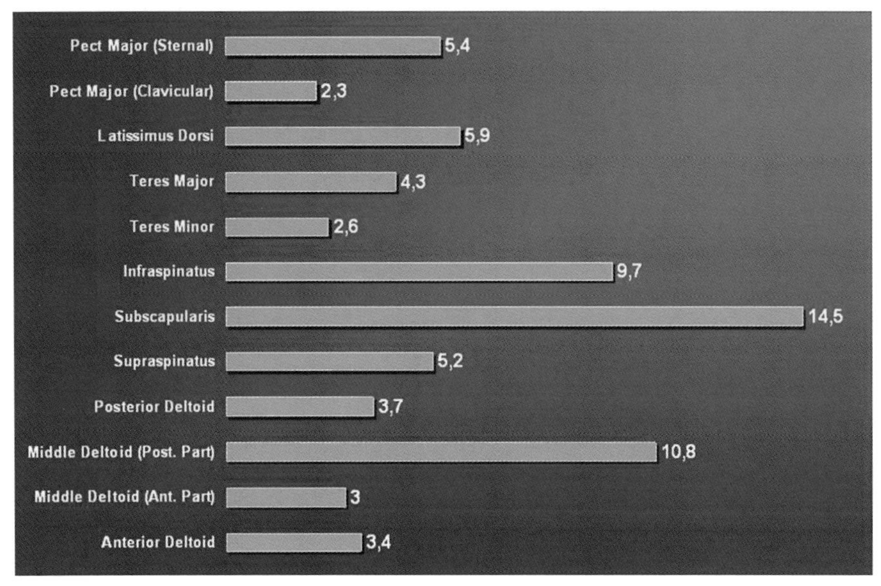

Fig. 5 – Our findings regarding the distribution of relative tension values (%) in 12 muscle bellies of the shoulder girdle that may be involved in tendon transfers, either as recipients or as donors. Note that the percentages values are expressed among the whole shoulder girdle muscles (21 muscle bellies).

Study of the point of fixation of latissimus dorsi MTT

Theoretical values of abduction/adduction and external/internal rotation moment arms of innate infraspinatus and latissimus dorsi MTT to either supraspinatus, infraspinatus, or teres minor footprints are shown in Figs. 6-8. Because of a deleterious bowstringing effect (with adduction torque) of the latissimus dorsi transfer when the humerus was in 60° internal rotation it was concluded that the best point of fixation was at the infraspinatus footprint (Fig. 9). According to our experiment and whatever the position of the humerus, this provided a good external rotation torque and some abduction torque as well (34).

Discussion

There are limitations to any biomechanical in vitro studies and this paper is not intended to give a cookbook about the choices and methods of MTT to treat irreparable rotator cuff tears. However, the orientation of muscle fibers within a muscle determines its function (32) and this important architectural factor was taken into account in our study. Additionally, the large number of shoulder muscles included in the current study makes comparisons possible.

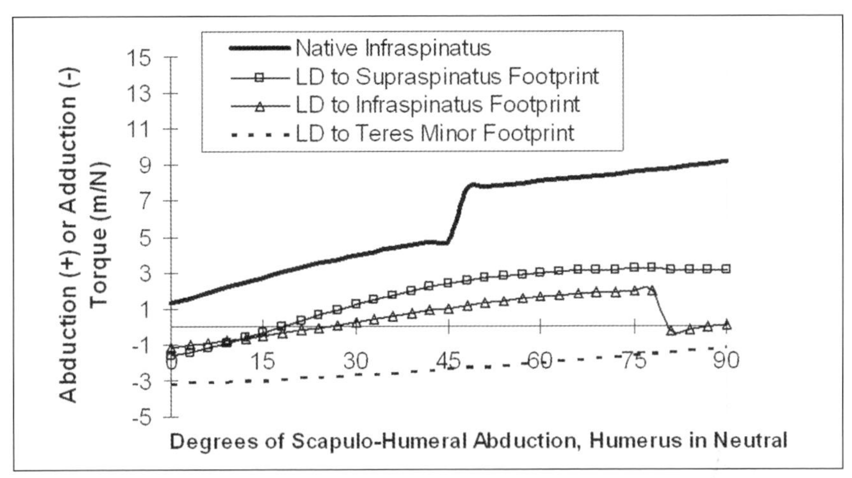

Fig. 6 – Abduction/adduction torque of native infraspinatus compared with latissimus dorsi transfer to supraspinatus, infraspinatus, or teres major footprints. Modelization of scapulo-humeral abduction at 3° increments is provided. Humerus is in neutral position relative to scapula, i.e., perpendicular to the plane of the scapula.

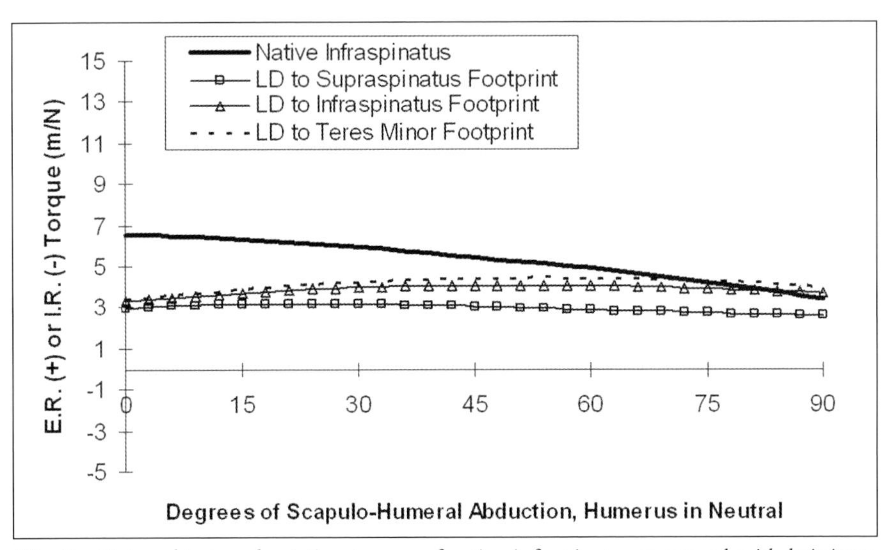

Fig. 7 – External/internal rotation torque of native infraspinatus compared with latissimus dorsi transfer to supraspinatus, infraspinatus, or teres major footprints. Modelization of scapulo-humeral abduction at 3° increments is provided. Humerus is in neutral position relative to scapula, i.e., perpendicular to the plane of the scapula.

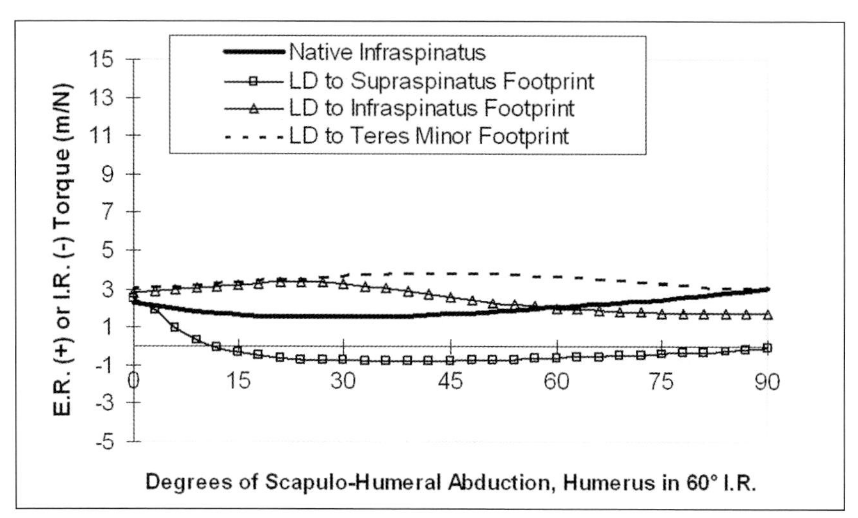

Fig. 8 – External/internal rotation torque of native infraspinatus compared with latissimus dorsi transfer to supraspinatus, infraspinatus, or teres major footprints. Modelization of scapulo-humeral abduction at 3° increments is provided. Humerus is in 60° internal rotation relative to scapula.

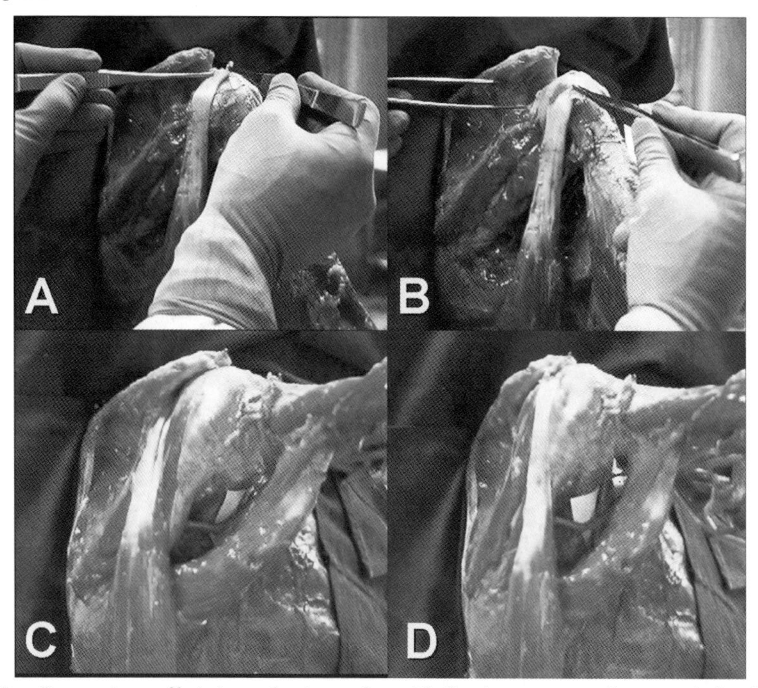

Fig. 9 – Comparison of latissimus dorsi transfers with fixation to supraspinatus or infraspinatus. (A) Fixation to supraspinatus insertion, (B) fixation to infraspinatus insertion, (C) fixation to supraspinatus insertion with humerus in abduction and internal rotation (note the bowstringing effect of the tendon, and compare with Fig. 8 showing deleterious internal rotation torque), and (D) fixation to infraspinatus insertion with humerus in abduction and internal rotation (external rotation torque is provided; compare with Fig. 8).

In a particular patient, muscle tension may be highly variable as exercise may strengthen a muscle in a few months, while joint disease may cause wasting. However, the relative muscle-to-muscle strength of a given group of muscles should remain fairly constant that makes the value of experimental comparative studies. Regarding the shoulder, this assumption is valid only in cadavers with an intact cuff; they have to be carefully selected among elderly cadavers because massive tears may induce hypertrophy of the teres minor muscle (37) and imply a significant bias. The possibility of compensatory hypertrophy of a muscle has been demonstrated experimentally after surgical removal or denervation of synergists (38).

Patients with irreparable cuff tears lost their normal shoulder girdle muscles synchronism and equilibrium. If a surgical indication is chosen (7), they require a restoration of their shoulder girdle muscles balance, provided that their glenohumeral cartilage is preserved. Most of the time, irreparable cuff tears are posterosuperior. In this situation, surgery should restore the balance of abductor muscles against adductors and gravity in order to get functional shoulder elevation. Surgery should also get functional external rotation by restoring the balance between external and internal rotator muscles. A functional external rotation will help shoulder elevation. This means that harvesting an adductor or an internal rotator muscle (as latissimus dorsi or teres major), i.e., removing an adductor and internal rotation force, is as important as reinforcing abduction and external rotation by that same muscle transferred to a new insertion. This provides a "rebalancing" of the muscles. This is probably why the weak transfers of latissimus dorsi and teres major provide useful clinical results, provided that the subscapularis remains intact (28) to maintain the internal/external rotation balance of the shoulder. The deltoid flap (39-41) is theoretically more questionable in terms of vectors because it removes an abductor muscle belly. Combination of transfers may be able to restore a new functional muscle balance to a shoulder presenting with irreparable rotator cuff tear (Fig. 10). In particular, adjunction of the teres major to the latissimus dorsi (24, 42-44) may further weaken the internal rotation forces and improve the strength of the transfer in terms of structural properties. Of course, the current status of all muscles of the shoulder girdle of any particular patient should be considered (45) because some muscles may be very atrophied but some others may be hypertrophied (6, 37) and each situation is specific. The limitation of MRI is that it provides a poor indication of muscle biomechanical properties because the orientation of the muscle fibers cannot be determined (46). For anterosuperior defects, the pectoralis major transfer (either taken as a whole or a part of it) removes an adductor and internal rotator in order to compensate for a deficient subscapularis (44, 47-54). Other combinations of MTT have also been proposed (55, 56).

Whatever the planned transfer to treat an irreparable rotator cuff tear, it is useful to have available a database of mechanical properties of the shoulder girdle muscles. This is why several studies have addressed this topic (33, 57-60). It is interesting to note that despite different experimental methods, several studies provided similar partial results (7, 61). Our study considered all muscles of the

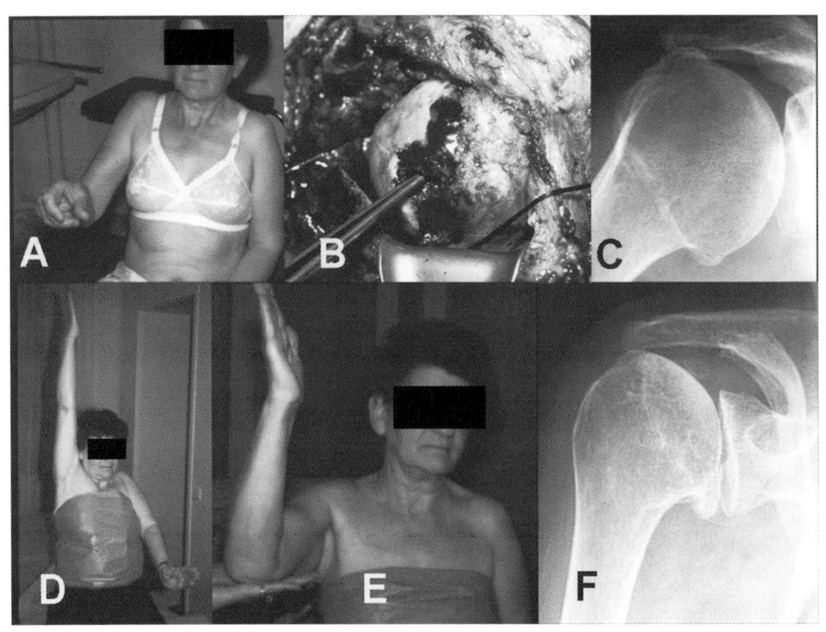

Fig. 10 – Why we should believe in tendon transfers to treat irreparable rotator cuff tears in selected patients? This 58-year-old female had pseudoparalytic shoulder (A) from a massive irreparable (B) rotator cuff tear of her right shoulder with shortened acromio-humeral distance and early glenohumeral arthritis. She was operated on with combined latissimus dorsi, teres major transfers, and deltoid flap. Result at 20 years follow-up in abduction (D) and external rotation at side (E). Note that the left shoulder was paralyzed due to sequellae of obstetrical brachial plexus palsy. Radiographs at 20 years follow-up showing marked progression of glenohumeral arthritis. This patient's was painless however, with a 74 pts constant score.

shoulder girdle and our results regarding rotator cuff muscles PCSA are consistent with other studies (57, 59). Thus it may be useful to consider this database and the muscles removed versus the muscles transferred before embarking in a shoulder rebalancing to treat an irreparable rotator cuff tear. Of course many other factors (13, 62) are to be considered, including patient's psychomotor skills (29) and compliance. We have shown that surgical technique is also very important in order to avoid excessive tension on the pedicles of the transferred muscle(s) after surgery (63). Another critical point is how the MTT should be set at surgery in terms of passive stretching. Although the knowledge of the theoretical Blix curve of the MTT according to shoulder muscle databases (33) is valid to set the transfer at a proper tension, i.e., close to its resting length, objective methods are lacking for optimal "tensioning" of a tendon transfer (46). About the point of fixation of the latissimus dorsi transfer, there are also limitations from this modelization, as others. However it was rather obvious from the graphs and video pictures (Fig. 9A-D) that transferring the latissimus dorsi too anteriorly may create a deleterious bowstringing effect during shoulder abduction for a small amount of internal rotation of the humerus. The take-home message of this particular work is to think of and avoid a possible bowstringing effect in internal rotation of the humerus when a very anterior point of distal fixation on the humerus is chosen for the latissimus dorsi. Ideally, the point of fixation should remain lateral to the projection of the center of rotation of the humerus, irrespective of the shoulder position.

References

1. Gerber C, Vinh TS, Hertel R, Hess CW (1988) Latissimus dorsi transfer for the treatment of massive tear of the rotator cuff: a preliminary report. Clin Orthop; (232): 327-329
2. Aoki M, Okamura K, Fukushima S, Takahashi T, Ogino T (1996) Transfer of latissimus dorsi for irreparable rotator-cuff tears. J Bone Joint Surg (Br); 78 B(5): 761-766
3. Birmingham PM, Neviaser RJ (2008) Outcome of latissimus dorsi transfer as a salvage procedure for failed rotator cuff repair with loss of elevation. J Shoulder Elbow Surg; 17: 871-874
4. Boileau P, Chuinard C, Neyton L, Trojani C (2007) Modified LD and Teres major transfer through a single delto pectoral approach for external rotation deficit of the shoulder: as an isolated procedure or with a reverse arthroplasty. J Shoulder Elbow Surg; 16: 671-682
5. Codsi MJ, Williams GR, Iannotti JP. (2007) LD tendon transfer for irreparable posterosuperior rotator cuff tears. Surgical technique. J Bone Joint Surg Am; 89A(suppl. 2, part 1): 1
6. Costouros JG, Gerber C (2007) Teres minor integrity predicts outcome of LD tendon transfer for irreparable rotator cuff tears. J Shoulder Elbow Surg; 16: 727
7. Costouros JG, Gerber C, Warner JJP (2007) Management of irreparable rotator cuff tears: the role of tendon transfers. In: Iannotti JP, Williams GR, editors. Disorders of the shoulder. Philadelphia: Lippincott Williams & Wilkins: 101-146
8. Degreef I (2005) Treatment of irreparable rotator cuff tears by Latissimus Dorsi transfer. Acta Orthop Belg; 71: 667-671
9. Elhassan B, Warner JJP (2008) Transfer of pectoralis major for the treatment of irreparable tears of the subscapularis. Does it work? J Bone Joint Surg (Br); 90B: 1059
10. Gerber C (2006) Latissimus dorsi transfer for the treatment of irreparable rotator cuff teats. J Bone Joint Surg Am; 88A: 113
11. Gerber C, Hersche O (1997) Tendon transfers for the treatment of irreparable rotator cuff defects. Orthop Clin North Am; 28(2): 195-203
12. Habermeyer P (2006) Transfer of the tendon of latissimus dorsi for the treatment of massive tears of the rotator cuff; a new single incision technique. J Bone Joint Surg (Br); 88B: 208
13. Iannotti JP, Williams GR (2006) Latissimus dorsi tendon transfer for irreparable postero-superior rotator cuff tears; factors affecting outcome. J Bone Joint Surg Am; 88A: 342

14. Irlenbusch U (2008) EMG analysis of muscle function after LD tendon transfer. J Shoulder Elbow Surg; 17: 492
15. Irlenbusch U (2008) Latissimus dorsi transfer for irreparable rotator cuff tears: a longitudinal study. J Shoulder Elbow Surg; 17: 527-534
16. Jennings GJ (2007) Transfer of segmentally split pect major for the treatment of irreparable rupture of the subscapularis tendon. J Shoulder Elbow Surg; 16
17. Konrad GG, McMahon PJ (2007) Pectoralis major tendon transfers above or underneath the conjoint tendon in subscapularis deficient shoulders. An in vitro biomechanical analysis. J Bone Joint Surg Am; 89A: 2477
18. Lu XW, Gazielly DF (2008) Long term outcomes after deltoid muscular flap transfer for irreparable rotator cuff tears. J Shoulder Elbow Surg; 17: 732
19. Mansat M (1996) Place des lambeaux musculo-tendineux dans les ruptures irréparables de la coiffe des rotateurs de l'épaule. 8ème Cahier d'Enseignement de la Société Française de Chirurgie de la Main. Paris: Expansion Scientifique Française, 119-129
20. Miniaci A, MacLeod M (1999) Transfer of the latissimus dorsi muscle after failed repair of a massive tear of the rotator cuff. A two to five-year review. J Bone Joint Surg Am; 81A: 1120-1127
21. Morelli M, Miniaci A (2008) LD tendon transfer for massive irreparable cuff tears: an anatomic study. J Shoulder Elbow Surg; 17: 139
22. Moursy M, Resch H (2009) Latissimus dorsi tendon transfer for irreparable rotator cuff tears: a modified technique to improve tendon transfer integrity. J Bone Joint Surg Am 1924
23. Nové-Josserand L, Liotard JP, Walch G (2009) Résutats du transfert du latissimus dorsi pour rupture non reparable de la coiffe des rotateurs. Rev Chir Orthop; 95: 125-130
24. Pearle AD, Warren RF (2006) Surgical technique and anatomic study of Latissimus dorsi and teres major transfers. J Bone Joint Surg Am; 88A: 1524
25. Postacchini F (2002) Latissimus dorsi transfer for primary treatment of irreparable rotator cuff tears. J Orthopaed Traumatol; 2: 139-145
26. Warner JJP (2000) Management of massive irreparable rotator cuff tears: the role of tendon transfer. J Bone Joint Surg Am; 82A: 878-887
27. Warner JJP (2001) Latissimus dorsi tendon transfer: a comparative analysis of primary and salvage reconstruction of massive irreparable cuff tears. J Shoulder Elbow Surg; 10: 514-521
28. Werner CML, Gerber C (2006) The biomechanical role of the subscapularis in LD transfer for the treatment of irreparable rotator cuff tears. J Shoulder Elbow Surg; 15: 736
29. Werner CML, Gerber C (2008) Influence of psychomotor skills and innervation patterns on results of LD tendon transfer for irreparable RC tears. J Shoulder Elbow Surg; 17 (suppl. 1): 22S
30. Brand PW, Hollister A (1993) Clinical mechanics of the hand. 2nd ed. St Louis: Mosby

31. Lieber RL, Fazeli BM, Botte MJ (1990) Architecture of selected wrist flexor and extensor muscles. J Hand Surg; 15 A: 244-250
32. Brand PW, Beach RB, Thompson DE (1981) Relative tension and potential excursion of muscles in the forearm and hand. J Hand Surg; 6(3): 209-219
33. Herzberg G, Urien JP, Dimnet J (1999) Potential excursion and relative tension of muscles in the shoulder girdle: relevance to tendon transfers. J Shoulder Elbow Surg; 8: 430-437
34. Herzberg G, Berthonnaud E, Schoierer O, Guigual V, Dimnet J, Morin A (2001) Latissimus dorsi transfer in irreparable rotator cuff tears: what point of fixation on the humeral head? Orthop Trans
35. Minagawa H, Itoi E (1998) Humeral attachment of the supraspinatus and infraspinatus tendons: an anatomic study. Arthroscopy; 14(3): 302-306
36. Berthonnaud E, Herzberg G, Zhao KD, An KN, Dimnet J (2005) Three dimensional in vivo displacements of the shoulder complex from biplanar radiography. Surg Radiol Anat; 27: 214-222
37. Walch G (1998) The dropping and hornblower's signs in evaluation of rotator cuff tears. J Bone Joint Surg (Br); 80B: 624-628
38. Baldwin KM, Valdez V, Herrick RE, MacIntosh AM, Roy RR (1982) Biomechanical properties of overloaded fast-twitch skeletal muscle. J Appl Physiol; 52: 467-472
39. Augereau B, Vandenbussche E (1997) Deltoid flap in rotator cuff tears retracted to the glenoid rim. In: Gazielly DF, Gleyze P, Thomas T, editors. The Cuff. Paris: Elsevier: 356-359
40. Gazielly DF, Gleyze P, Verney-Carron J, Bruyère G, Montagnon C, Thomas T (1997) Deltoid muscle flap transfer for the treatment of chronic irreparable cuff tears. In: Gazielly DF, Gleyze P, Thomas T, editors. The Cuff. Paris: Elsevier: 361-365
41. Le Huec JC, Liquois F, Schaeverbecke T, Zipoli B, Chauveaux D, Le Rebeller A (1996) Résultats d'une série de lambeaux deltoidiens pour rupture massive de la coiffe des rotateurs avec 3,5 ans de recul moyen. Rev Chir Orthop; 82: 22-28
42. Berthonnaud E, Herzberg G, Schoierer O, Medda N, Dimnet J (2003) Latissimus dorsi transfer: should we add the teres major? Orthop Trans
43. Celli L (1998) Transplantation of teres major muscle for infraspinatus muscle in irreparable rotator cuff tears. J Shoulder Elbow Surg; 7: 485-490
44. Combes JM, Mansat M (1995) Traitement des ruptures massives de la coiffe des rotateurs par lambeau du muscle grand rond. Etude expérimentale. In: Bonnel F, editor. L'épaule musculaire. Montpellier: Sauramps Médical: 227-236
45. Lehtenin JT, Tingart MJ, Apreleva M (2003) Practical assessment of rotator cuff muscle volume using MRI. Acta Orthop Scand; 74: 722
46. Lieber RL (2008) Biology and mechanics of skeletal muscle: what hand surgeons need to know when tensioning a tendon transfer. JHSA; 33A: 1655
47. Galatz LM, Yamaguchi K (2003) Pectoralis major transfer for anterior-superior subluxation in massive rotator cuff insufficiency. J Shoulder Elbow Surg; 12: 1-5

48. Jost B, Gerber C (2003) Outcome of pectoralis major transfer for the treatment of irreparable subscapularis tears. J Bone Joint Surg Am; 85A: 1944-1951
49. Jost B, Gerber C (2004) Pectoralis major transfer for subscapularis insufficiency. Techniques in Shoulder and Elbow Surgery; 5: 157
50. Klepps S, Yamaguchi K (2001) Subcoracoid pectoralis major transfer: a salvage procedure for irreparable subscapularis deficiency. Tech Shoulder Elbow Surg; 2: 85-91
51. Resch H (2000) Transfer of the Pectoralis major muscle for the treatment of irreparable rupture of the subscapularis tendon. J Bone Joint Surg Am; 82A: 372-382
52. Resch H (2002) Pectoralis major muscle transfer for irreparable rupture of the subscapularis and supraspinatus tendon. Tech Shoulder Elbow Surg; 3: 167-173
53. Vidil A, Augereau B (2000) Le lambeau du chef claviculaire du grand pectorel dans les ruptures irréparables du subscapulaire. Rev Chir Orthop; 86: 835-843
54. Wang AA, Strauch RJ, Flatow EL, Bigliani LU, Rosenwasser MP (1999) The teres major muscle: an anatomic study of its use as a tendon transfer. J Shoulder Elbow Surg; 8: 334-338
55. Gerber A, Warner JJP (2004) Split pectoralis major and teres major tendon transfers for reconstruction of irreparable tears of the subscapularis. Tech Shoulder Elbow Surg; 5: 5-12
56. Mack Alridge J, Atkinson TS, Mallon WJ (2004) Combined pectoralis major and LD tendon transfer for massive rotator cuff deficiency. J Shoulder Elbow Surg; 13: 621-629
57. Bassett RW, Browne AO, Morrey BF, An KN (1990) Glenohumeral muscle force and moment mechanics in a position of shoulder instability. J Biomechanics; 23(5): 405-415
58. Bonnel F (1995) Les muscles de l'épaule. Equilibre stato-dynamique. Morphologie. Biométrie. In: Bonnel F, editor. L'épaule musculaire. Montpellier: Sauramps Médical: 33-76
59. Keating IF, Waterworth P, Shaw-Dunn J (1993) The relative strength of the rotator cuff muscles. J Bone Joint Surg (Br); 75B: 137
60. McMahon PJ, Debski RE, Thompson WO, Warner JJP, Fu FH, Woo SLY (1995) Shoulder muscle forces and tendon excursions during glenohumeral abduction in the scapular plane. J Shoulder Elbow Surg; 4: 199-208
61. Magermans DJ (2004) Biomechanical analysis of tendon transfers for massive rotator cuff tears. Clin Biomech; 19: 350-357
62. Goutallier D (2004) Table Ronde: le traitement chirurgical des ruptures associées des supra épineux et infra épineux non réparables par simple suture. Rev Chir Orthop; 90 (suppl au n° 5): IS154
63. Schoierer O, Herzberg G, Berthonnaud E, Dimnet J, Aswad R, Morin A (2001) Anatomical basis of Latissimus dorsi and teres major transfers in rotator cuff tear surgery with particular reference to the neurovascular pedicles. Surg Radiol Anat; 23: 75-80

Latissimus dorsi transfer for massive and irreparable rotator cuff tears

J. Garret, J. Kany, C. Lévigne, H.A. Kumar, S. Grosclaude

The latissimus dorsi muscle is the pillar of reconstructive surgeries around the shoulder and the chest. It is widely used in the breast reconstruction, for covering large musculo-cutaneous defects either as free flap or with neuro-vascular pedicle.

It can be used for dynamic active restoration of flexion or extension of the elbow. Around the shoulder, the transferred latissimus dorsi muscle serves for restoration of external rotation either primarily or in revision procedure for massive and irreparable cuff tears.

Indications for surgery (Fig. 1 with four slides)

The latissimus dorsi transfer (LDT) is indicated in irreparable and massive posterosuperior rotator cuff tears with deficit in active external rotation of the shoulder (1).

The LDT is contraindicated in case of deltoid dysfunction (primarily, or due to previous surgeries) (2, 3), and in case of associated subscapularis tears (1, 3, 5).

In posterosuperior rotator cuff tear, symptoms are loss of active external rotation and associated shoulder pain. Pain intensity is variable and prominently during the night. The active external rotation of the shoulder varies from a simple drop force to a pseudoparalytic shoulder. A chronic pseudoparalytic shoulder may be a contraindication to the transfer for some (13, 14) authors. Age is not a prognosis factor (10). Patients may have multiple surgeries for the shoulder, with sometimes several failed attempts to repair the rotator cuff. Salvage procedure is a bad prognostic factor for this transfer (10).

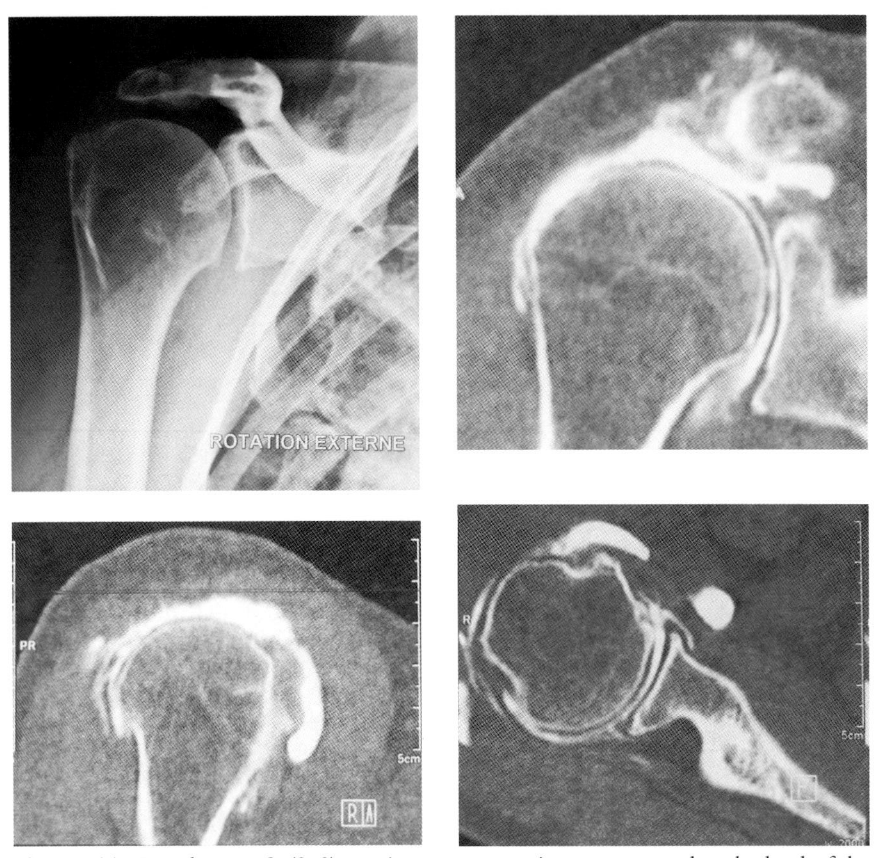

Fig. 1 – (1) Hamada stage 2, (2, 3) massive posterosuperior tear retracted at the level of the glenoid, good subscapularis, and (4) supraspinatus and infraspinatus tear with atrophic muscle and fatty infiltration >3 (Goutallier classification).

The external rotation power is graded into six grades according to the international classification (MRC grading), in positions RE1 and RE2:

M0: no contracture
M1: obvious contracture without movement
M2: partial movement against gravity
M3: complete movement against gravity
M4: complete movement against weak degree of resistance
M5: complete movement against resistance of moderate degree

Several clinical signs exist to estimate the degree of loss in active external rotation:

(1) The "lag sign" (6) measures the degree of loss of active external rotation RE1 with regards to contralateral side of the body.
(2) The dropping sign (7) is an automatic return to the neutral rotation of the hand of the patient that is placed in maximal external rotation by

the examiner. In more severe cases, the hand automatically returns to the stomach of the patient. A positive sign indicates tear of infraspinatus.

(3) The hornblower (7) sign represents the inability for the hand to reach the mouth without raising up the elbow. It indicates the association of teres minor tear along with the supraspinatus and infraspinatus tears.

The other clinical examination verifies the absence of deltoid and active internal rotation. The "lift off test" and the "belly press test" are normal.

The standard radiological assessment includes three different views of the glenohumeral joint (in neutral, internal, and external rotations). This allows the Hamada's classification for the cuff tear arthropathy to be applied (8). The results of the LDT are proportional to the preservation of the subacromial space. Hamada stages 4 and 5, where there is a glenohumeral degenerative osteoarthrosis, are contraindicated. The prediction outcomes are also poor in stage 3 with complete pinching and "acetabulization" of the acromion.

Arthro-CT or arthroMRI or MRI assess stage of tendon retraction and quality of muscles (atrophy and fatty infiltration). Muscle fatty infiltration may be stage by the classification of Goutallier and al. (12).

Operative technique

The latissimus dorsi is a flat muscle with 38 cm length, 20 cm width, and about 0.8 cm thickness. It takes its origin from the apophyses of the T6 to L5, the sacrum, and the iliac crest. The musculo-tendinous unit rotates around itself 180° to insert on the medial border of the bicipital groove on the proximal humerus.

The muscle is vascularized by a main pedicle, the artery is a branch from the subscapularis artery. There is a single vein accompanying the thoraco-dorsal artery. The thoraco-dorsal artery penetrates the latissimus dorsi muscle at 10 cm below the humeral insertion and 2 cm from the lateral border of the muscle.

The innervation of the latissimus dorsi muscle is from the thoraco-dorsal nerve originating from the posterior cord of the brachial plexus. This joins the vascular pedicle to penetrate the muscle belly along with them.

Step 1 (Fig. 2)

Superior deltoid splitting approach to proximal humerus is preferred; for this purpose the patient is positioned in decubitus 30° and with posterior tilt of 30°. This position optimally allows for the superior deltoid splitting and exposure of the proximal humerus for the harvesting of latissimus dorsi tendon simultaneously. The ruptured cuff tendons can also be visualized at the same time.

The various procedures are:
- subacromial bursectomy, acromioplasty;
- greater tuberositoplasty;
- tenotomy or tenodesis of the biceps tendon into the bicipital groove;
- partial repair of the cuff muscles if possible.

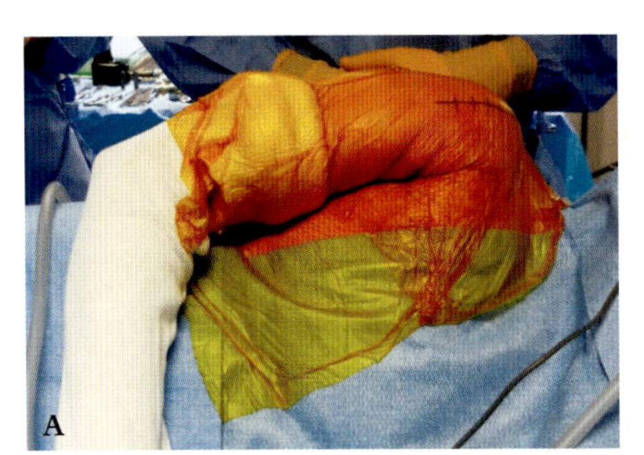

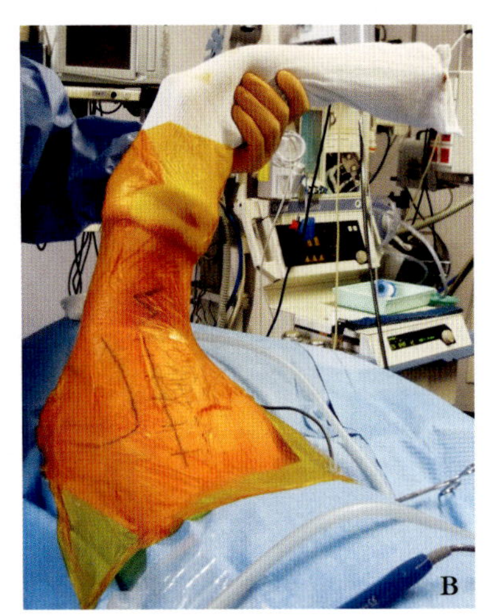

Fig. 2 – (A) Anterosuperior approach, (B) axillary approach to harvest and to release latissimus dorsi from the angle of the scapula.

Step 2: Harvesting the tendon of latissimus dorsi (Fig. 3)

The incision is made along the lateral boarder of the latissimus dorsi muscle on the scapular border extended above till the axillary hollow to prevent any retractile scar. Dissecting in the subcutaneous plan the latissimus dorsi is released from all superficial adhesions. The lateral boarder and the apex of the scapula are identified. It is important to spend some time in dissecting clearly the boarders of latissimus dorsi and teres major. There is a fatty demarcation between these two muscles. It is necessary to separate these two muscles and to release all the adhesions from the undersurface of the latissimus dorsi till the apex of the scapula, because this determines the excursion of the transferred tendon. The deeper adhesions are easy to remove. The freed muscle is raised and reclined backwards allowing the exposure of the thoraco-dorsal pedicle.

We expose the tendon of the latissimus dorsi until its insertion on the humerus, inner border of the bicipital groove. The shoulder is positioned in abduction and maximal internal rotation at this point. The tendon is sectioned in contact with the humerus in order to achieve the maximum length possible.

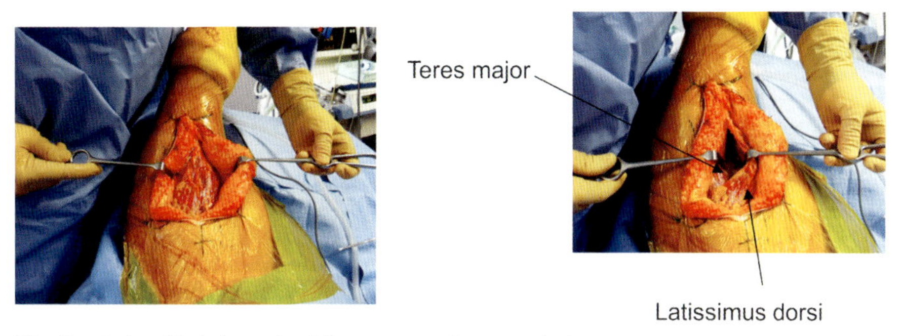

Fig. 3 – Isolated latissimus dorsi from teres major posteriorly.

Step 3: Tubulization of the tendon and tunnelization under the deltoid (Figs. 4 and 5)

The latissimus dorsi tendon is a flat. Tunnelization is realised from posterior to anterior under the deltoïd. It has to be very careful and driven behind the long head of the triceps and the axillary pedicle.

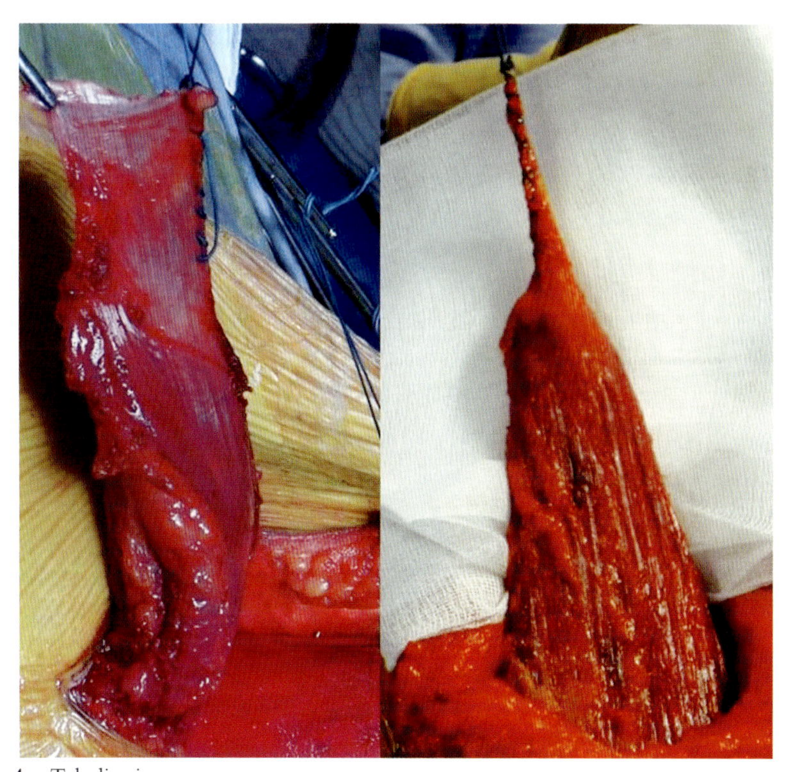

Fig. 4 – Tubulization.

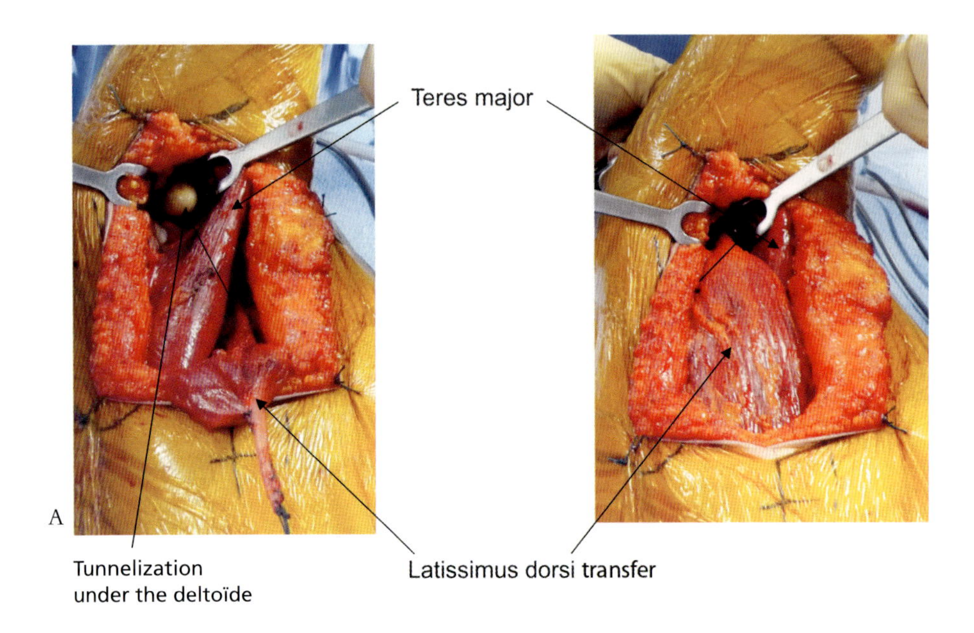

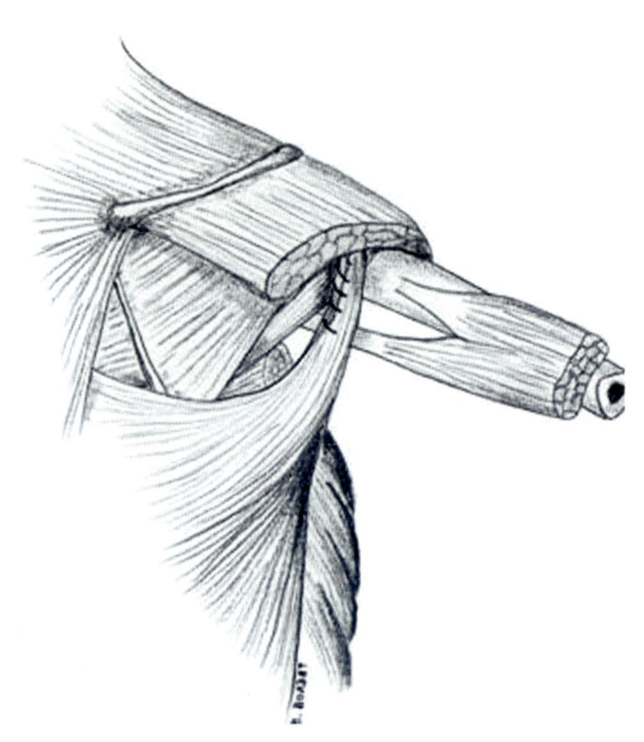

Fig. 5 – (A) Tunnelization of latissimus dorsi and (B) tunnelization of latissimus dorsi under the posterior deltoid (Illustration by courtesy of the Dr Bertrand Bordet, Clinique du Parc, Lyon, France).

Step 4: Fixation of the latissimus dorsi into the transosseous tunnel of remplace made in the greater tuberosity (Fig. 6)

The transosseous tunnel is realized in the greater tuberosity at the junction of the insertion of supraspinatus and infraspinatus tendon in the direction of the bicipital groove. The tunnel is prepared to appropriate size as the diameter of the latissimus dorsi tendon previously measured with graded drilling. In most of the cases, the diameter is 7 mm.

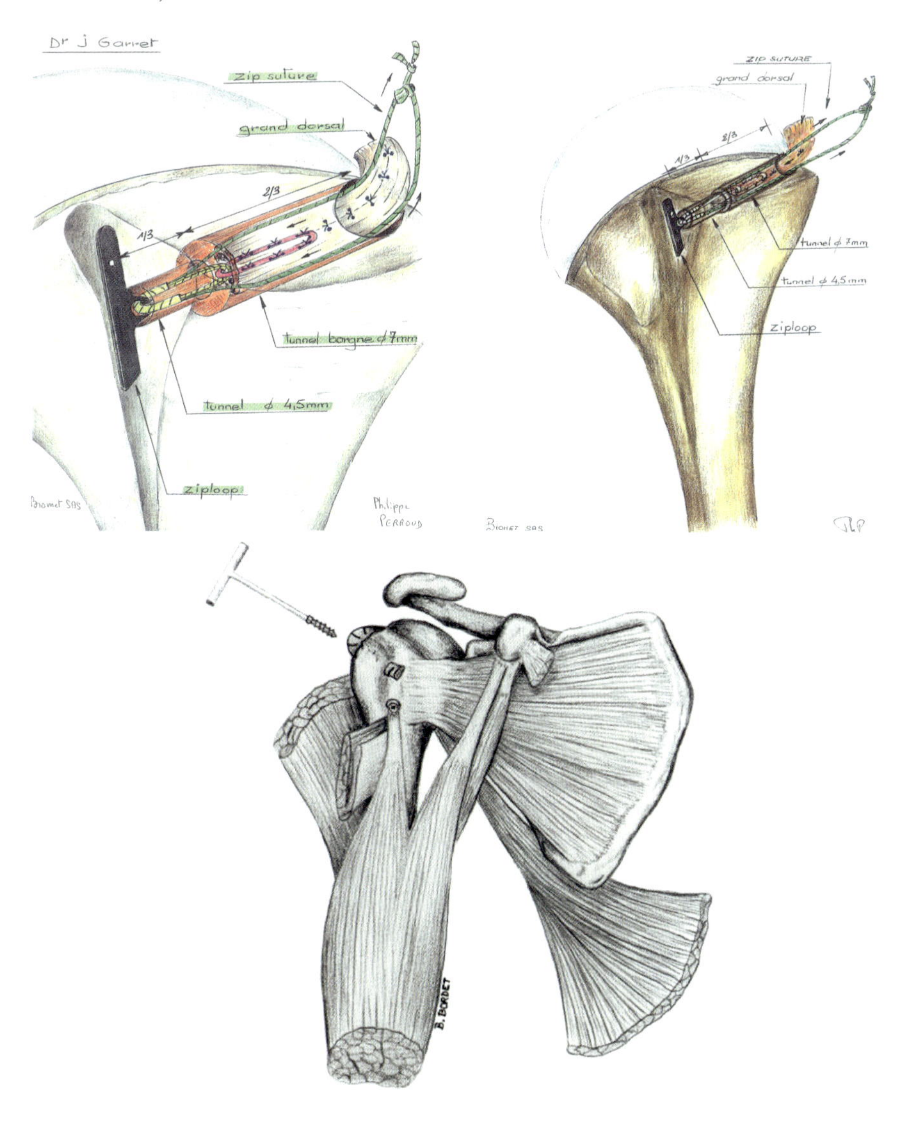

.../...

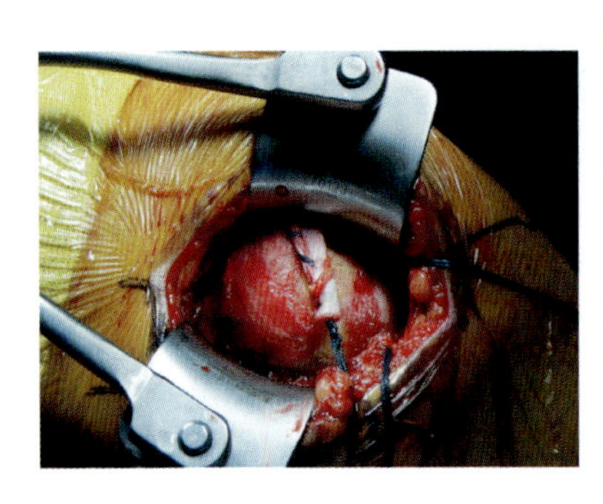

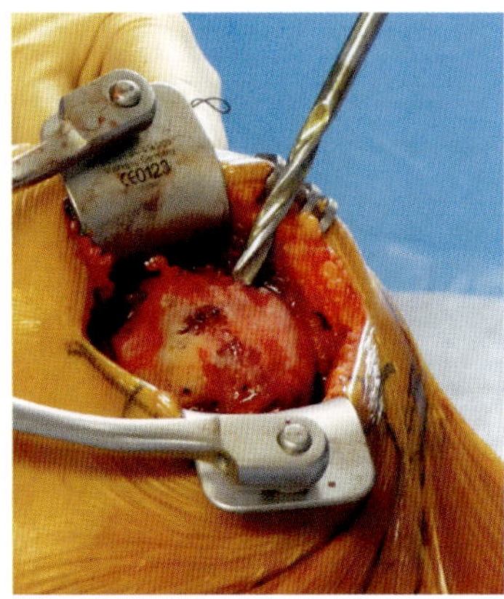

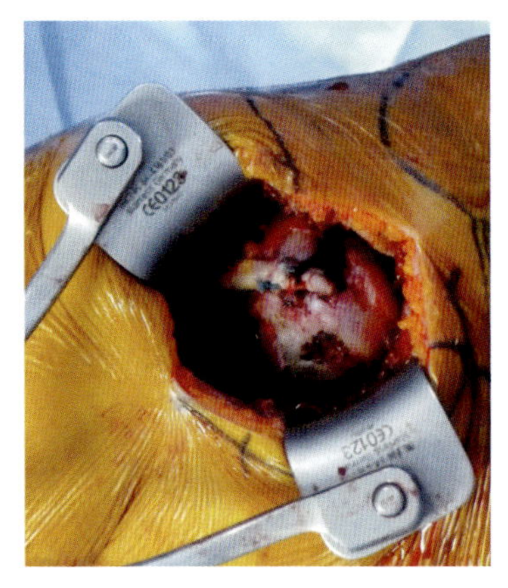

Fig. 6 – Tubulization of the latissimus dorsi and fixation with a Zip Loop TM (Biomet Inc.) at the level of the footprint between the area of insertion of supraspinatus and infraspinatus tendon. (Third illustration by courtesy of the Dr Bertrand Bordet, Clinique du Parc, Lyon, France).

The tendon is then introduced into the osseous tunnel with the help of suture threads attached earlier. The transfer is fixed in the position of maximum tension with arm abduction of 60° and in neutral rotation. Its fixation has been described using multiple anchors or transosseous interference screw. We propose to secure it with special endobutton Zip Loop TM (biomet Inc.). This device allows solid fixation with maximum tension on the transfer tendon which is in our view a key factor of success.

The closure of the wound is done in layers with a suction drain in situ. The patient is immobilized in a splint pillow of abduction 60°. The passive mobilization is started immediately with the help of physiotherapist. The immobilization is continued for 6-8 weeks.

The daily life activities may be started after 3 months.

References

1. Gerber C, Vinh TS, Hertel R, Hess CW (1988) Latissimus dorsi transfer for the treatment of massive tears of rotator cuff. A preliminary report. Clin Orthop; 232: 51-61
2. Miniaci A, Macleod M (1998) Transfer of latissimus dorsi muscle after failed repair of massive tear of the rotator cuff. A two to five year review. J Bone Joint Surg; 81A: 1120-1127
3. Postacchini F, Gumina S (2002) Results of surgery after failed attempt at repair of irreparable rotator cuff tear. Clin Orthop Relat Res; 397: 332-341
4. Gerber C, Maquiera G, Espinosa N (2006) Latissimus dorsi transfer for the treatment of irreparable rotator cuff tears. J Bone Joint Surg; 88A: 113-120
5. Werner CM, Zing PO, Lie D, Jacob, HA, Gerber C (2006) The biomechanical role of the subscapularis in latissimus dorsi transfer for the treatment of irreparable rotator cuff tears. J Shoulder Elbow Surg; 15: 736-742
6. Hertel R, Ballmet FT, Lombert SM, Gerber C (1996) Lag sign in diagnostis of rotator cuff rupture. J Shoulder Elbow Surg; 5: 307-313
7. Walch G, Boulahia A, Calderone S (1998) The "dropping" and the "hornblower" signs in evaluation of rotator cuff tears. J Bone Joint Surg; 80B: 624-628
8. Hamada K, Fukuda H, Mikasa M, Kobayashi Y (1990) Roentgenographic findings in massive rotator cuff tears. A long term observation. Clin Orthop Relat Res; 254: 92-96
9. Gerber C (1992) Latissimus dorsi transfer for treatment of irreparable tears of rotator cuff. Clin Orthop; 275: 152-160
10. Nové Josserand L, Costa P, Liotard JP, Safar JF, Walch G, Zilber S (2009) Results of latissimus tendon transfer for irreparable cuff tears. Orthop Traumatol: Surg Res; 95: 108-113
11. Patte D (1990) Classification of rotator cuff lesion. Clin Orthop Relat Res
12. Goutallier D, Postel JM, Bernageau J, Lavau L, Voisin MC (1994) Fatty muscle degeneration in cuff ruptures. Pre and postoperative evaluation by CT scan. Clin Orthop Relat Res; 304: 78-83
13. Iannotti JP, Hennigan S, Herzog R, Kella S, Kelley M, Leggin B, et al. (2006) Latissimus dorsi tendon transfer for irreparable postero-superior rotator cuff tears. Factors affecting outcome. J Bone Joint Surg; 88A: 342-348
14. Codsi MJ, Hennigan S, Herzog R, Kella S, Kelley M, Leggin B, et al. (2007) Latissimus dorsi tendon transfer for irreparable posterosuperior rotator cuff tears. Surgical technique. J Bone Joint Surg; 89A (suppl. 2): 1-9

Results of latissimus dorsi tendon transfer in primary or salvage reconstruction of massive, irreparable rotator cuff tears

Ph. Valenti, I. Kalouche, L.C. Diaz, A. Kaouar, A. Kilinc

Introduction

Irreparable rotator cuff rupture is defined as the inability to reattach the cuff tendons on the greater tuberosity despite a release of the deep and superficial parts of cuff (1); it may be associated with persistent pain and functional disability.

Several methods have been proposed to restore active elevation of the shoulder after anterior irreparable rupture of the rotator cuff, most of which gave random results such as synthetic implants (2), deltoid flap (3), and the translation of the upper subscapularis (4). The transfer of the latissimus dorsi proposed for the first time in 1988 by Gerber et al. (5) seems to yield better results. The flap helps stabilize the humeral head and then potentiates the action of the deltoid to enhance forward elevation. It also improves external rotation by its posterolateral angle of attack.

The aim of this retrospective study was to assess the results of the proposed technique as well as a first-line treatment and as a second option after failure of previous surgery in irreparable ruptures of the rotator cuff.

Materials and methods

This is a retrospective, monocentric study, covering 25 consecutive patients with massive irreparable rotator cuff rupture treated with an isolated transfer of the latissimus dorsi with a minimum follow-up of 1 year. The indication was a painful shoulder associated with a limitation of active anterior elevation (AAE) of 90° and a significant loss of strength. Patients with signs of a blow horner sign who were operated by a double transfer of the latissimus dorsi and teres major according to L'Episcopo (6), and those with a pseudoparalytic shoulder associated with an anterosuperior instability of a massive rupture of the rotator cuff were excluded from this study.

There were 14 men and 11 women with a mean age of 55.8 years (range 42-64 years). Seventeen patients had a latissimus dorsi transfer as a first-line surgery (group I) and 8 patients had this transfer as a second line after failure of previous surgery (group II). This latter group consisted of arthroscopic debridement in three cases and repair of the rotator cuff in five cases (open in three cases and under arthroscopy in two cases).

Twenty patients were manual workers. There were 15 cases of workplace accident. Trauma was present in only nine patients. All patients had received at least 30 rehabilitation sessions, which allowed them to improve the AAE but with persistent pain and an impingement. The symptoms most often associated pain, limited AAE (90°), and decreased strength.

Clinical examination found signs of anterosuperior and posterosuperior conflict in almost all cases. The palm-up test was positive in 17 patients showing pain of the long head of biceps. The lift-off test of Gerber was found in only one case. No patient had signs of horn blower prior to the operation that indicates a functional teres minor.

No patient had a deltoid's atrophy. We considered that the presence of a functional deltoid was a necessary condition for achieving the transfer of the latissimus dorsi.

Plain anteroposterior X-ray with the forearm in neutral rotation showed ascension of the humeral head in 20 cases. There still remains an acromiohumeral distance of at least 2-3 mm. The acromion was type I in 7 cases, type II in 14 cases, and type III in 4 cases according to Bigliani's classification (7). In one case, early glenohumeral osteoarthritis was noted.

The CT arthrogram found a rupture of supraspinatus and infraspinatus in 21 cases, rupture of the supraspinatus and subscapularis in 1 case, and a rupture of the three tendons in 2 cases. Lesions of the subscapularis interested less than half of the tendon in the sagittal plane. An isolated rupture of the infraspinatus was found in one case. The site of rupture is given in Table I. All ruptured tendons were retracted to the glenoid (stage 3). The index of average preoperative fatty degeneration according to Goutallier's classification (8) was 3.28 for the supraspinatus and the infraspinatus, and 0.6 for the subscapularis.

Surgery was done under general anesthesia and regional interscalenic block in all cases with patients in lateral position. A first lateral approach in front of the middle part of the acromion was done to assess the rotator cuff's rupture. The incision was started behind the acromio-clavicular joint, and was extended distally toward the middle deltoid without exceeding 4 cm above the lower edge of the acromion to avoid injury to the axillary nerve (Fig. 1).

Table I – Distribution of ruptures in the two groups.

	Supraspinatus and infraspinatus	*Supraspinatus and subscapularis*	*Supraspinatus, infraspinatus and subscapularis*	*Infraspinatus*
Group I	14	1	1	1
Group II	7	0	1	0
Total	21	1	2	1

Group I: first intention surgery; group II: secondary surgery.

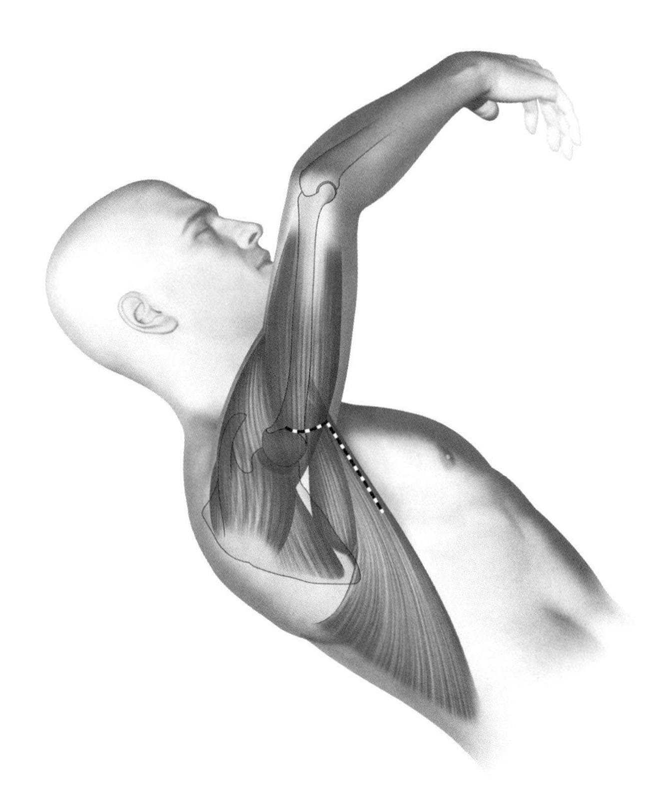

Fig. 1 – In beach chair position, axillary approach to harvest latissimus dorsi muscle.

A trapezo-deltoid flap was raised with chips of cancellous bone from acromion reducing the risk of detachment of the middle deltoid and facilitating its reinsertion. The coraco-acromial ligament was preserved to avoid weakening of the anterior part of the acromion that was already thinned in the middle and outer part. The long portion of the biceps tendon was preserved when it appeared unaltered (six cases) and fixed (tenodesis) in the bicipital groove (seven cases) or cutted (six cases) when it was subluxated or alterated.

In six cases it was previously ruptured. The harvesting of the latissimus dorsi was done through an axillary approach (Fig. 2). An incision of about 10 cm length was done at the anterior part of the latissimus dorsi and extended from the scapular angle toward the posterior part of the deltoid with a hook in the axilla, to avoid any scar contracture source of elevation limitation. The flap was separated from the teres major (not taken) posteriorely and from the serratus anterior in front and down from the fibrous subcutaneous and fibrous attachments at the angle of the scapula (Fig. 3). This release of the vasculo-nervous

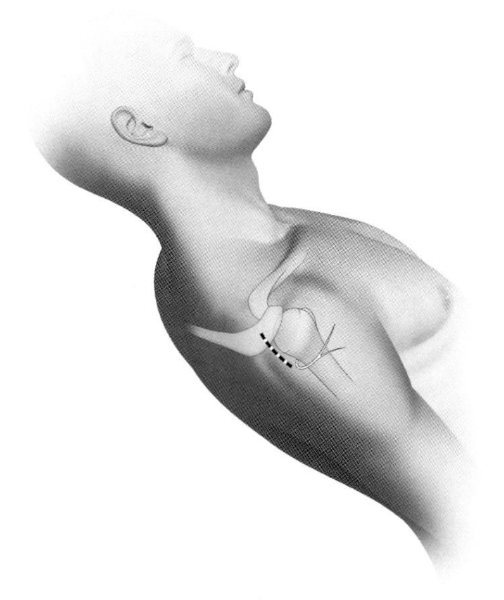

Fig. 2 – Anterosuperior transdeltoid approach.

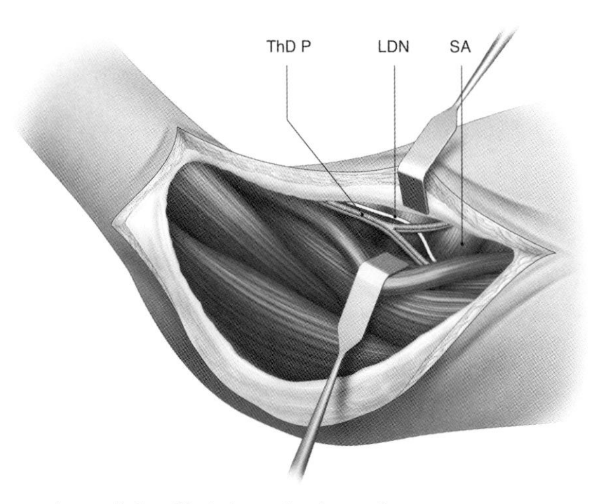

Fig. 3 – Neurovascular pedicle of latissimus dorsi muscle.
ThD P: Thoracodorsal pedicle; LND: Latissimus dorsi nerve; SA: Serratus anterior muscle.

pedicle (which is not dissected but simply visualized during dissection of the anterior aspect of latissimus dorsi) is essential for upper displacement of the flap without traction and fixation of the aponevrotic blade of the latissimus dorsi over the greater tuberosity (Fig. 4). The absence of release can put the sutures under tension with a flip of the scapula during abduction of the arm by tenodesis effect and a high risk of secondary dropping. The exposure and release of the aponevrotic fascia of the latissimus dorsi from the humerus requires a perfect knowledge of the radial nerve and axillary nerve whose position relative to the latissimus dorsi is variable depending on the rotation of the arm (Fig. 5). This anatomy has been well documented by the anatomical studies of Cleeman et al. (9) and Pearle et al. (10): the radial nerve is located at the bottom and front at an average distance of 2.9 cm while the axillary nerve is located more proximally at an average distance of 1.4 cm. No intraoperative lesion or postoperative deficit was found in the series. The aponevrotic fascia of the latissimus dorsi was desinserted with a large periosteum from the medial border of the humerus while positioning the arm in internal rotation. The fascial strip was passed under the posterior deltoid (Fig. 6) and posterior to the teres minor and then fixed on the greater tuberosity (insertion zone of the infraspinatus and supraspinatus) previously sharpened with at least four anchors for a large contact surface (Figs. 7 and 8). Suturing the stump of the cuff was done whenever it was possible (13 times out of 25 in our series). We found that positioning over the greater tuberosity was easier when the patient was slender: "stocky" and brachimorphic patients, with a large muscle and short course, do not represent a favorable anatomy for this type of surgery. But we try to fix it anteriorly if we want to restore AAE or more posteriorly at the level of the insertion of the infraspinatus if we want to restore external rotation (Figs. 9 and 10).

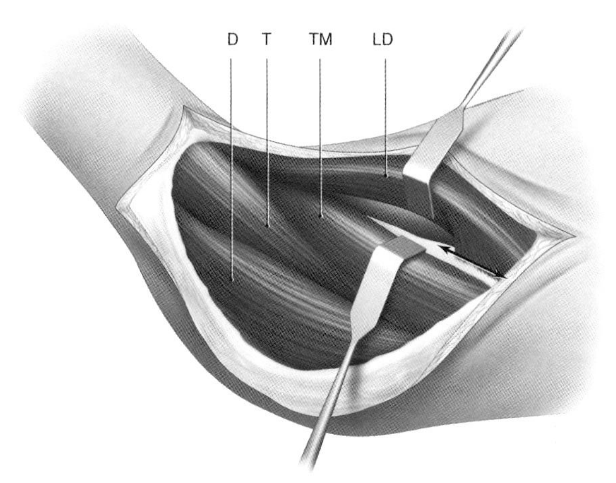

Fig. 4 – Release of latissimus dorsi from the teres major posteriorly, from the serratus anterior anteriorly, and from the angle of the scapula inferiorly.
D: Deltoid muscle; T: Triceps; TM: Teres major; LD: Latissimus dorsi.

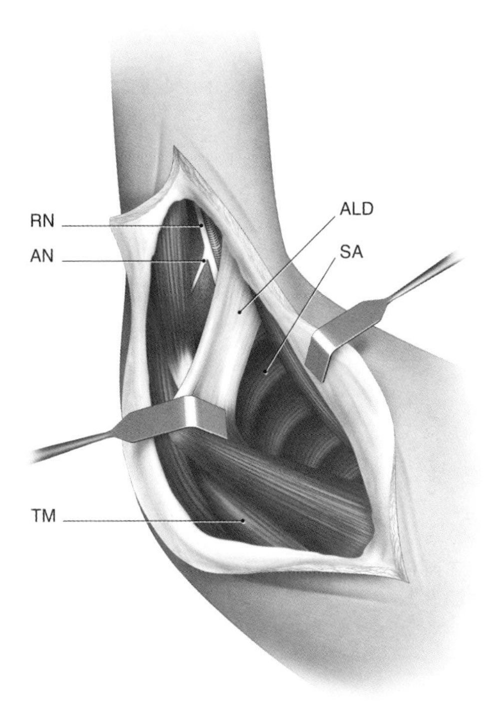

Fig. 5 – Dissection of the aponevrosis band of latissimus dorsi.
AN: Axillary nerve; RN: Radial nerve; TM: Teres major; ALD: Aponeurosis latissimus dorsi; SA: Serratus anterior.

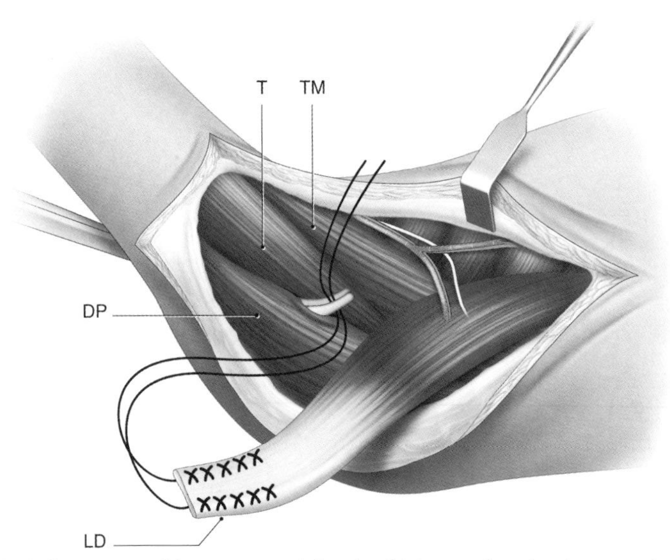

Fig. 6 – Reinforcement of the aponevrosis band, which passed under the posterior deltoid to the humeral head.
TM: Teres major; T: Triceps; DP: Deltoid posterior; LD: Latissimus dorsi.

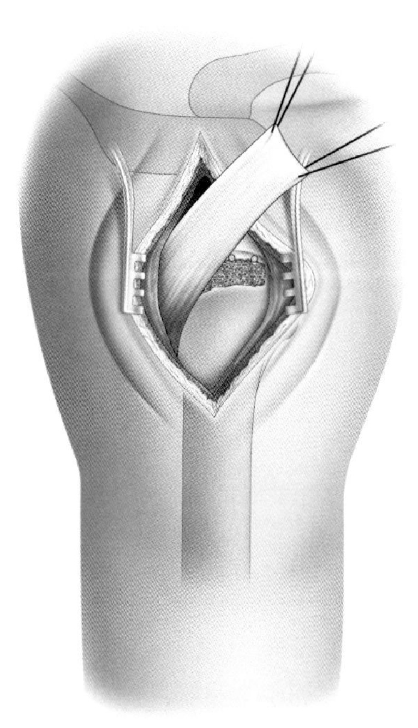

Fig. 7 – Fixation to the footprint abrased.

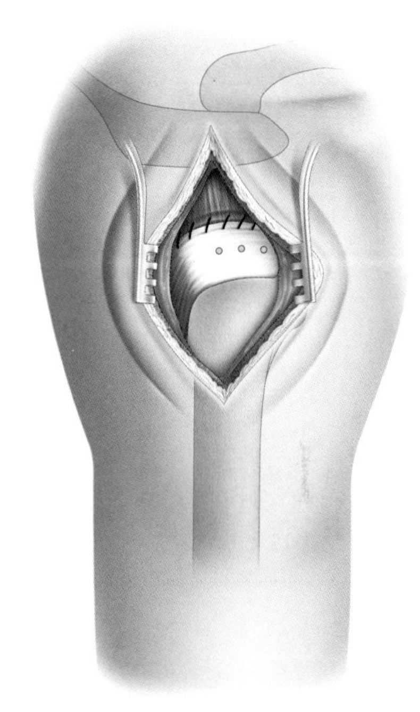

Fig. 8 – Fixation to a large area to facilitate tendon healing.

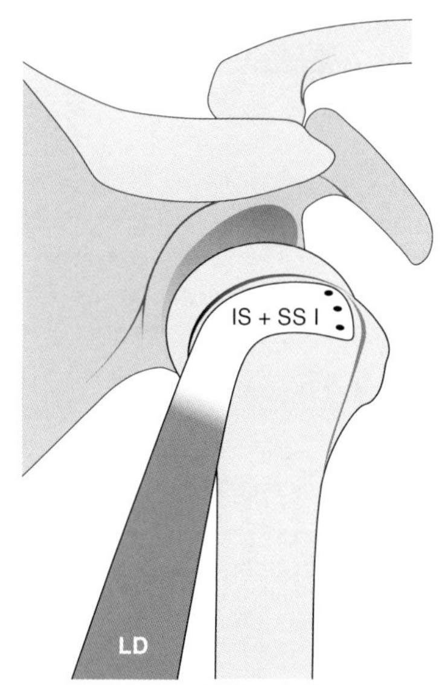

Fig. 9 – Fixation at the level of the supraspinatus to restore active elevation. IS + SS I: Infraspinatus + supraspinatus insertions; LD: Latissimus dorsi.

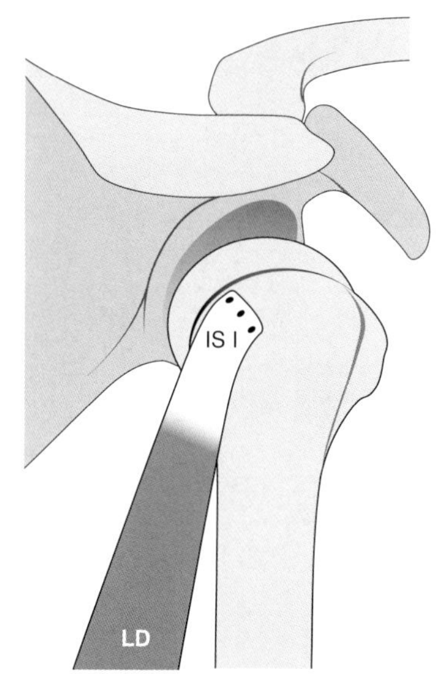

Fig. 10 – Fixation at the level of the infraspinatus to restore external rotation. IS I: Infraspinatus insertions; Ld: Latissimus dorsi.

Postoperative immobilization in 30° of abduction and 20° of external rotation was kept during 6 weeks. Passive mobilization was begun immediately and active mobilization at 6 weeks. The aim of physiotherapy was to restore an active external rotation and anterior elevation. The total duration of this physiotherapy was 6 months on average.

At the final follow-up, subjective assessment based on the degree of satisfaction and persistence or not of pain or functional impairment was performed, and objective assessment was based on active and passive joint mobilities and muscle strength. Absolute Constant and Murley score (11) was also calculated to assess gains in elevation and external rotation.

Statistical tests

The statistical tests used were Student's *T*-test when two groups were compared. Where there were more than two groups for comparison, analysis of variance was performed. The level of significance (p) was set at 0.05.

Results

No major complication (neurologic or infectious) was noted in this serie; two patients presented axillarie retractile scar that necessitated extended massage.

Results were appreciated at a mean follow-up of 22 months (range 12-60 months).

Mean AAE progressed from 94.4° to 151.6°, with a mean gain 57.2° (60.5%). This gain was significant ($p < 0.0001$). It was more important when the preoperative AAE was low. For patients with preoperative AAE less than 80°, the average gain was 82.5° (123%) against 18° (12%) for patients with preoperative AAE more than 120° (Table II). This difference between groups was significant ($p < 0.05$).

When comparing the two groups defined in 'materials and methods' section, the gain in AAE was higher in group I than in group II (Table III), however this difference was not statistically significant.

A significant gain of about 50% was obtained in external rotation. External rotation elbow to the body (ER1) increased from an average of 24.4° preoperatively to 36.4° after surgery ($p < 0.05$) and external rotation at 90° of abduction (ER2) from 33.2° to 50.4° ($p < 0.0001$).

As for AAE, the gain in external rotation was greater in patients with preoperative AAE less than 80 (Table I) and for patients in group I (Table II) but these differences were not significant.

Force has progressed very little from 3 points in pre-op to 5.12 after surgery without significant difference between the two groups I or II.

Table II – Results based on the preoperative AAE.

	AAE ≤ 80°	80° < AAE ≤ 120°	AAE > 120°
Nbr	12	8	5
AA E pre-op	66.6°	102°	148°
AAE post-op	149.1°	146.2°	166°
Gain AAE	82.5*	43.8	18*
ER1 pre-op	16.6°	21.2°	48°
ER1 post-op	31.6°	31.2°	56°
Gain ER1	15	10	8
ER2 pre-op	25.8°	28.5°	58°
ER2 post-op	42.5°	45°	78°
Gain ER2	16.6	16.3	20
CST pre-op	27.4	36.8	51.4
CST post-op	57.3	54.4	65.2
Gain CST	29.9*	16.8	13.8

AAE: anterior active elevation; pre-op: preoperative; post-op: postoperative; CST: absolute Constant score; Nbr: number of cases; *significant difference between groups, $p < 0.05$.

There was no significant difference in external rotation when the aponevrotic fascia was sutured or not to the rotator cuff stump (13 times out of 25).

The average absolute Constant score increased from 35.5 preoperatively to 58 after surgery, with a gain of 63.4%. This increase is significant ($p < 0.0001$). The largest gain was found for pain (89%), followed by activity (86%), strength (70%), and mobility (47%). Improvement in Constant score was higher for patients with preoperative AAE less than 80°. They have had an average gain of 30 points or 109%, against 16.8 points (47.5%) for patients with AAE between 80° and 120° and 13.8 points (26.8%) for patients with AAE more than 120° (Table I). However, only the difference in gain between the group of patients with preoperative AAE less than 80° and the group with preoperative AAE higher than 120° was statistically significant. Similarly, the gain was greater for patients in group I for which the Constant score increased from 35.8 preoperatively to 60.8 after surgery realizing a gain of 25 points from 70% against 49% for patients in group II: this difference was not statistically significant.

The gain in Constant score was improved when fatty degeneration was less than 4 with a gain of 91% against only 49% when fatty degeneration was 4 without being significant ($p < 0.08$).

Table III – Results based on surgical indication (first-line surgery: group I or second-line surgery: group II).

Group	I	II
Nbr	17	8
AA E pre-op	95,8°	91.2°
AAE post-op	159.4°*	135°*
Gain AAE	63.5°, 63.2%	43.8°, 48%
ER1 pre-op	24.1°	25°
ER1 post-op	39.4°*	30°
Gain ER1	15.3°, 63.4%	5°, 20%
ER2 pre-op	31.2°	37.5°
ER2 post-op	52.4°*	46.3°
Gain ER2	21.2°, 68%	8.7°, 23.2%
CST pre-op	35.8	34.9
CST post-op	60.8*	51.9*
Gain CST	25.1, 68%	17, 38.7%

AAE: anterior active elevation, pre-op: preoperative, post-op: postoperative, CST: absolute Constant score, Nbr: number of cases, *significant difference compared to preoperative values with $p < 0.05$.

At the final follow-up, 84% of patients were satisfied or very satisfied, 8% were somewhat satisfied and 8% consider it a failure. This subjective result is independent of age, sex, and a possible connection with a work accident. Otherwise, if the intervention was proposed as second line (group II), 50% of patients had subjective outcome as fair or poor. There was no difference in group II depending on the nature of previous surgery.

The lesion of the subscapularis tendon, involving only the upper half (confirmed intraoperatively) present in three patients in our study did not influence significantly the objective and subjective outcome. Indeed, these patients showed gains in active motion (active elevation: 82.5-157.5°, external rotation 1: 25-42.5°, and external rotation 2: 35-60°) and Constant score (30-58.5).

Discussion

The treatment of irreparable rotator cuff's rupture, particularly in younger patients, remains a difficult therapeutic challenge and choice of techniques is fairly limited. The successful use of the latissimus dorsi flap to restore elevation and external rotation in the sequelae of obstetrical paralysis of the brachial plexus (12-14) prompted Gerber et al. (5) to use this technique since 1988 for the irreparable rupture of the supraspinatus and infraspinatus. The successful results of this transfer in terms of pain, anterior elevation, and external rotation in posterosuperior lesions with an effective subscapularis reported by the latter in 1992 by Gerber (1) have allowed the extension of its use. Since then, several studies have been published (15-17) reporting equivalent results with this technique, which prove its reproducibility and biomechanical basis. The flap of the latissimus dorsi has a dual function: by its depressor and external rotation effects on the humeral head, it stabilizes and refocuses this latter and thus potentiates the action of elevation and abduction of the deltoid (15, 17). Thus the presence of an effective deltoid was a prerequisite for the realization of this tendon transfer (5). This was mentioned by several authors (16, 18) who consider that the deltoid muscle atrophy is a contraindication to the transfer of the latissimus dorsi. However, Miniaci and MacLeod (15) found no difference in outcomes in the presence or absence of lesions in the deltoid and concluded that the presence of competent deltoid is not absolutely necessary to realize the transfer.

The average postoperative AAE in our series was 151.6° with an average gain of 57.2°. This is in agreement with results reported by Gerber et al. (5) with a gain of 52° and slightly higher than the gain of 36° reported by Aoki et al. (17).

In the series of Warner and Parsons (16) comparing the results after primary surgery to those of the second-line surgery, postoperative AAE was 122° with an average gain of 60° for group I and 105° with a gain of 43° average for the second group. These gains are equivalent to those reported in our series. However, Miniaci and MacLeod (15) reported a gain of 57.8°, much higher in case of secondary surgery. Gerber et al. in 2006 (19) state that gains in indolence and mobility are similar in the two groups unless the patient who already had a shoulder surgery had a decrease in range of motion of his shoulder for a long time.

In our series, the gain in external rotation was 12° in ER1 from 24.4° to 36.4°. These results are equivalent to those found in the same study by Miniaci and MacLeod (15). However, the difference in gain between groups I and II (15.3 and 5) is not significant, which joins the results of the series of Warner and Parsons (16) where no difference between the two groups were noted in terms of external rotation.

In the series of Gerber et al. (5), the gain in Constant score was 73%; it was 63.3% in our series. In the series of Warner and Parsons (16), the postoperative Constant score was 69 for group I with a gain of 33%, and 52 for group II with a gain of 16%. Better gain was noticed in our series for each group, but the Constant scores remain lower than those found by Warner and Parsons (16). This is because the preoperative score in the series of Warner is higher than in our series.

Moreover, the Constant score does not exceed more than 60 points. This score is lower than what is found after a conventional repair (open or arthroscopic) of the cuff that provides a Constant score between 81 (20) and 84 (21). Patients should be cautioned that the expected functional recovery is lower than that obtained after a conventional repair of the rotator cuff. According to Warner and Parsons (16), lack of information is responsible for most of the iterative ruptures of the tendon transfer, especially in cases of significant immediate improvement. The clinical outcome determined at the end of the first year has not deteriorated with the follow-up (for patients with a long follow-up), which could mean the absence of iterative rupture in our series, however, no postoperative electromyogram was done to confirm the evidence that the transfer contracts and no MRI has been able to analyze the presence of the fascial strip on the greater tuberosity in our series.

In our study, 84% of patients were very satisfied or satisfied. This is in agreement with the results reported by Gerber et al. (5), Aoki et al. (17), and Miniaci and MacLeod (15) with respectively 80%, 75%, and 82% excellent and good results. In the series of Warner and Parsons (16), equivalent results were obtained for group I (83% of cases). For group II in our series as in that of Warner, 50% of patients had an average or bad score.

The influence of the integrity of the subscapularis on the results of this transfer remains controversial. A biomechanical study conducted by Werner et al. (22) highlighted the role of the subscapularis in stabilizing the humeral head in the transverse plane. Its absence or disability would be responsible for anterior subluxation of the humeral head. In the original series of Gerber, the Constant score in overall was 73 at the follow-up and increased to 83 after exclusion of patients with lesions of the subscapularis. Warner and Parsons (16) and Codsi et al. (18) reported that the rupture of the subscapularis is a contraindication for the transfer of latissimus dorsi; on the other hand, Miniaci and MacLeod (15) think that it is not a factor of poor prognosis.

The low number of cases of rupture of the subscapularis (three cases) involving the upper half does not allow us to conclude about the absolute contraindication of the latissimus dorsi flap. However the association of an anterior transfer of teres major fixed on the lower part of the lesser tuberosity could replace the action of the missing subscapularis and thus improve the effectiveness of the latissimus dorsi (it was done twice with good results; patients are not included in this series).

Costouros et al. (23) showed that fatty infiltration of the teres minor more than 2 regarding Goutallier classification is a negative predicting factor in outcome of latissimus dorsi tendon transfer. We did not evaluate all the patients of our series and we are not able to conclude a correlation between status of teres minor and outcome of latissimus dorsi tendon transfer.

In this current study, with a too short follow-up (12-60 months), loss of acromio-humeral distance and increasing of glenohumeral arthritis, as showed by Gerber et al. (19), were not noted.

The inferior results of a second-line surgery in comparison to surgery of first line could have many explications.

The role of preoperative fatty degeneration has been demonstrated by Warner and Parsons (16) who found that the results were worse when the preoperative fatty degeneration was important. In our series, the degree of fatty degeneration did not affect significantly the absolute result.

The role of the deltoid injury is quite controversial. Thus, although most authors emphasize the harmful effect of these lesions caused primarily by surgery prior to transfer, Miniaci and MacLeod (15) did not reveal any objective difference in the final outcome by presence or non-presence of such lesions.

In our study, prognosis was much better when the preoperative AAE was diminished. Codsi et al. (18) feel that the significant decrease of preoperative mobility including the AAE is a factor of poor prognosis and an AAE less than 80° preoperatively is a relative contraindication.

In conclusion, according to this study, the transfer of the latissimus dorsi is a surgical technique useful if the cuff repair is not possible with conventional techniques such that all treatment options are very limited in this situation. We reserve the transfer of isolated latissimus dorsi to the posterosuperior lesions with a functional subscapularis. The tendon transfer can reduce pain and improve the previous elevation and external rotation, and these gains are more significant when the deficit was important prior to the operation. However it is a rescue procedure and patients should be cautioned that these results are lower than those obtained after repair of the rotator cuff, especially if the transfer follows a first repair attempt.

The prognostic factors are difficult to identify precisely, but we still believe that it is necessary to have a competent deltoid to expect a satisfactory AAE. The revision surgery could be a factor of poor prognosis. Furthermore, the role of the subscapularis, the fatty degeneration, and the possibility of suturing the stump of the cuff remain controversial. A prospective study may clarify these factors.

References

1. Gerber C (1992) Latissimus dorsi transfer for the treatment of irreparable tears of the rotator cuff. Clin Orthop Relat Res; 275: 152-160
2. Ozaki JF, Fugimoto S, Masuhara K (1984) Repair of chronic massive rotator cuff tears with synthetic fabrics. In: Repair of chronic massive rotator cuff tears with synthetic fabrics. Philadelphia: Decker BC: 185-191
3. Apoil A, Augereau B (1985) Deltoid flap repair of large losses of substance of the shoulder rotator cuff. Chirurgie; 111 (3): 287-290
4. Cofield RH (1982) Subscapular muscle transposition for repair of chronic rotator cuff tears. Surg Gynecol Obstet; 154 (5): 667-672

5. Gerber C, Vinh TS, Hertel R, Hess CW (1988) Latissimus dorsi transfer for the treatment of massive tears of the rotator cuff. A preliminary report. Clin Orthop Relat Res; 232: 51-61
6. L'Episcopo JB (1934) Tendon transplantation on obstetrical paralysis. Am J Surg; 25: 122-125
7. Bigliani LU, Morrison DS, April EW (1986) The morphology of the acromion and its relationship to rotator cuff tears. Orthop Trans; 10: 228
8. Goutallier D, Postel JM, Bernageau J, Lavau L, Voisin MC (1994) Fatty muscle degeneration in cuff ruptures. Pre- and postoperative evaluation by CT scan. Clin Orthop Relat Res; 304: 78-83
9. Cleeman E, Hazrati Y, Auerbach JD, Shubin Stein K, Hausman M, Flatow EL (2003) Latissimus dorsi tendon transfer for massive rotator cuff tears: a cadaveric study. J Shoulder Elbow Surg; 12 (6): 539-543
10. Pearle AD, Kelly BT, Voos JE, Chehab EL, Warren RF (2006) Surgical technique and anatomic study of latissimus dorsi and teres major transfers. J Bone Joint Surg Am; 88 (7): 1524-1531
11. Constant CR, Murley AH (1987) A clinical method of functional assessment of the shoulder. Clin Orthop Relat Res; 214: 160-164
12. Wickstrom J, Haslam ET, Hutchinson RH (1955) The surgical management of residual deformities of the shoulder following birth injuries of the brachial plexus. J Bone Joint Surg Am; 37A (1): 27-36; passim
13. Hoffer MM, Wickenden R, Roper B (1978) Brachial plexus birth palsies. Results of tendon transfers to the rotator cuff. J Bone Joint Surg Am; 60 (5): 691-695
14. Gilbert A, Tassin JL, Benjeddou MS (1978) Paralysie obstetricale du membre superieur. Encycl Med Chir, Pédiatrie. Elsevier
15. Miniaci A, MacLeod M (1999) Transfer of the latissimus dorsi muscle after failed repair of a massive tear of the rotator cuff. A two to five-year review. J Bone Joint Surg Am; 81 (8): 1120-1127
16. Warner JJ, Parsons IMT (2001) Latissimus dorsi tendon transfer: a comparative analysis of primary and salvage reconstruction of massive, irreparable rotator cuff tears. J Shoulder Elbow Surg; 10 (6): 514-521
17. Aoki M, Okamura K, Fukushima S, Takahashi T, Ogino T (1996) Transfer of latissimus dorsi for irreparable rotator-cuff tears. J Bone Joint Surg Br; 78 (5): 761-766
18. Codsi MJ, Hennigan S, Herzog R, Kella S, Kelley M, Leggin B, Williams GR, Iannotti JP (2007) Latissimus dorsi tendon transfer for irreparable posterosuperior rotator cuff tears. Surgical technique. J Bone Joint Surg Am; 89 (suppl. 2, part 1): 1-9
19. Gerber C, Maquieira G, Espinosa N (2006) Latissimus dorsi transfer for the treatment of irreparable rotator cuff tears. J Bone Joint Surg Am; 88 (1): 113-120
20. Gazielly DF, Gleyze P, Montagnon C (1994) Functional and anatomical results after rotator cuff repair. Clin Orthop Relat Res; 304: 43-53

21. Levy O, Venkateswaran B, Even T, Ravenscroft M, Copeland S (2008) Mid-term clinical and sonographic outcome of arthroscopic repair of the rotator cuff. J Bone Joint Surg Br; 90 (10): 1341-1347
22. Werner CM, Zingg PO, Lie D, Jacob HA, Gerber C (2006) The biomechanical role of the subscapularis in latissimus dorsi transfer for the treatment of irreparable rotator cuff tears. J Shoulder Elbow Surg; 15 (6): 736-742
23. John G. Costouros, Norman Espinosa, Marius R (2007) Schmid, Christian Gerber. Teres minor integrity predicts outcome of latissimus dorsi tendon transfer for irreparable rotator cuff tears. J Shoulder Elbow Surg; 16 (6): 727-734

Arthroscopic humeral head interference screw fixation for latissimus dorsi transfer in massive and irreparable posterosuperior cuff tear

J. Kany, H.A. Kumar, J. Garret, Ph. Valenti

Introduction

Thirty percent of the patients attending shoulder specialty centers for surgery present with the challenge of massive and irreparable rotator cuff tears (1). Some of these patients have already been operated by open or arthroscopic technique, even before the age of 50 years. Gerber et al. (2) are the first to publish flap surgery for the treatment of these massive and irreparable cuffs. They cautioned about the indications of this LD flap when posterosuperior cuff tears were associated with subscapularis tears as the results were guarded and disappointing. Other authors (3-5) also confirmed poor results in case of subscapularis tears, deltoid anterior deficit, and as salvage procedure, where no solution exists today.

It is surprising that till date no publication has revealed the technical difficulties for fixation of such important transfer onto a bone of bad quality. One can suture the tendon directly to the subscapularis, transosseous bone sutures, or multiple classical anchors (6-10). Constantly, great tuberosity is fragile due to previous surgery or lack of mechanical stimulus chronically by the absence of cuff.

We hypothesized that failures of this transfer were also due to lack of adequate strong and stable fixation of the LD tendon onto the greater tuberosity. From the experience of the ACL reconstruction of the knee, as well as from the work of Boileau et al. (11) in the tenodesis of long head of biceps into the humeral head, we describe a new technique of fixation of the latissimus dorsi tendon by tubularization and interference screw into a bone tunnel made at the top of the humeral head. This technique, initially performed by open procedure, now switched to arthroscopic procedure that prevents a new deltoid damaging surgical approach.

Classic operative technique: direct IFS

Axillary dissection of the transfer was first described by Jérôme Garret.

The use of preoperative Echo-Doppler can be helpful in precise identification of the pedicle of the latissimus dorsi for easy intraoperative identification by causing less trauma to the pedicle by blind exploration and a mini invasive incision around the pre-marked pedicle on the skin.

It is fundamental to look for the maximum length of the tendon. One has to internally rotate the shoulder and place a Howman retractor more proximally around the diaphysis. Then dissection can be done from the periosteum to gain about 2 cm extra length of the tendon.

Before tenotomy, we advise to put two 4 cm sutures apart in the muscle belly on either side of the pedicle to assess the maximum physiological tension in abduction and internal rotation. The same tension will be applied during the fixation of the transfer into the humeral head (Fig. 1).

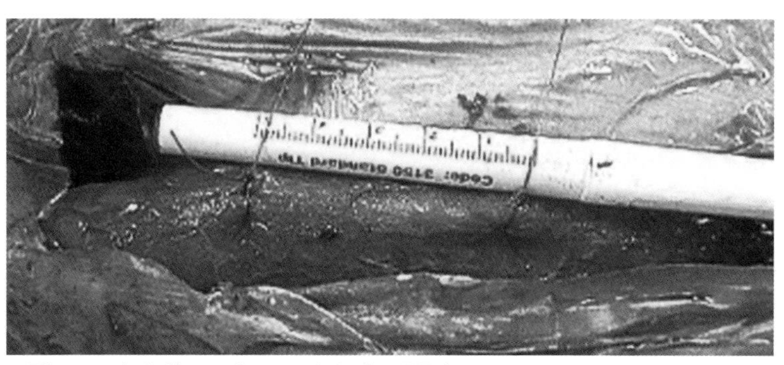

Fig. 1 – The muscle belly tension repair before LD humerus tenotomy.

Tenotomy will be done proximally (near the circumflex vessels) to distally, where there is no risk. It is important to be cautious regarding the deep big axillary vessels few centimeters medially. Once detached, the tendon is brought outside for tubularization (Fig. 2). A well-dissected tendon measures about 7 cm in length. The tendon itself is a long and flat structure that can be tubularized like semitendinous for ACL reconstruction. The average diameter after tubularization is about 7 mm (Figs. 3 and 4). Then, it is easy to release the muscle belly from the inconstant fibrous bands beneath itself and the apex of the scapula. After complete successful release, it should be easy to pass fingers all around the muscle belly without any difficulty. This gives good length for the tendon to be mobilized till the top of humeral head.

The pedicle must remain without any impingement throughout the entire process.

The tendon is passed behind the triceps but in front of the posterior deltoid as close as possible from the posterior surface of great tuberosity. The tendon is fixed onto the top of the humeral head near the junction of articular

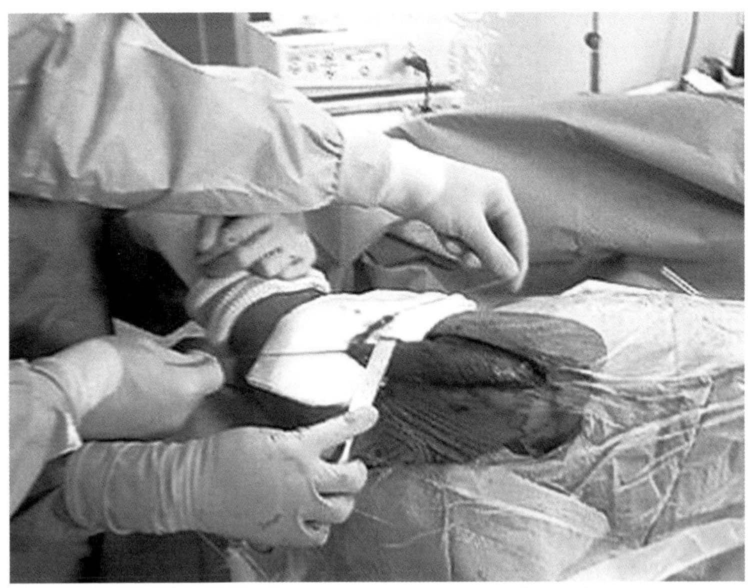

Fig. 2 – Two tractions sutures used to penetrate arthroscopically the bone tunnel.

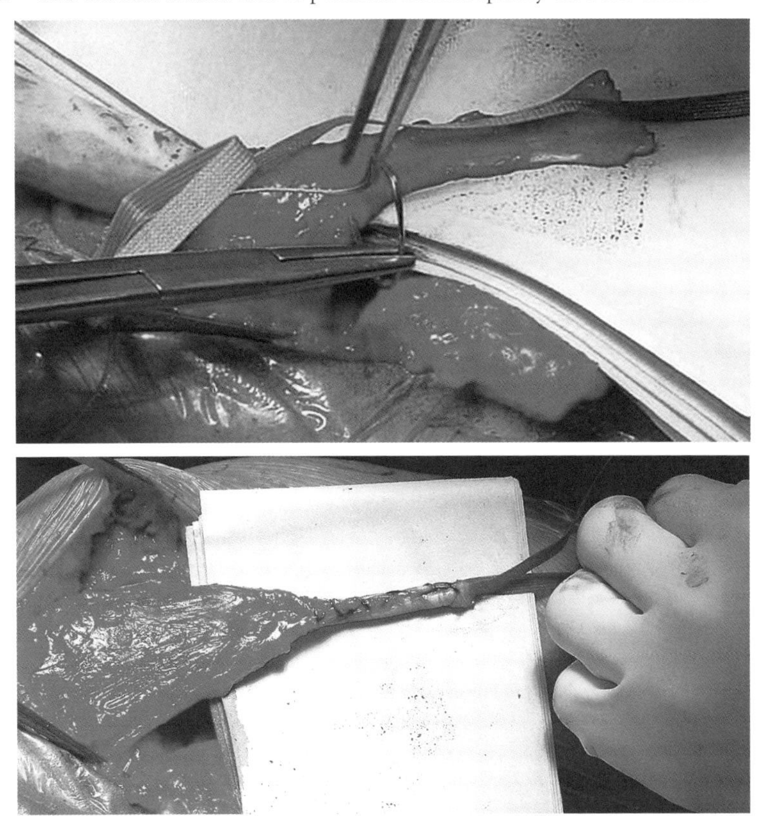

Figs. 3 and 4 – Tubulization of latissimus dorsi.

cartilage, to pass above the center of rotation of the shoulder. This transfer will be effective in external rotation and forward flexion. This transfer will also be effective in humerus head lowering. It is possible to fix it onto the posterior surface of the great tuberosity: this insertion will give more external rotation, but less forward flexion.

An ACL guide can be useful to find the good way out. It is advisable to use the Neviaser portal when required (over-coverage lateral acromion shape).

The fixation of the transfer was done initially by open technique and later shifted to arthroscopy as our experience increased.

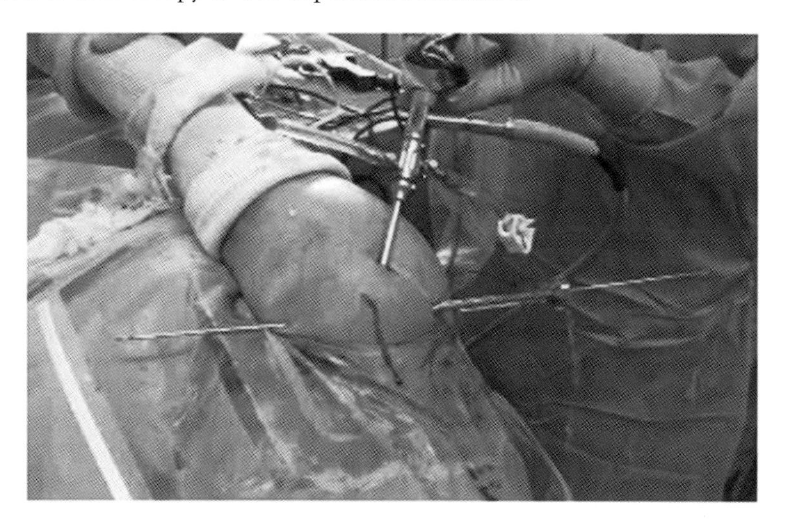

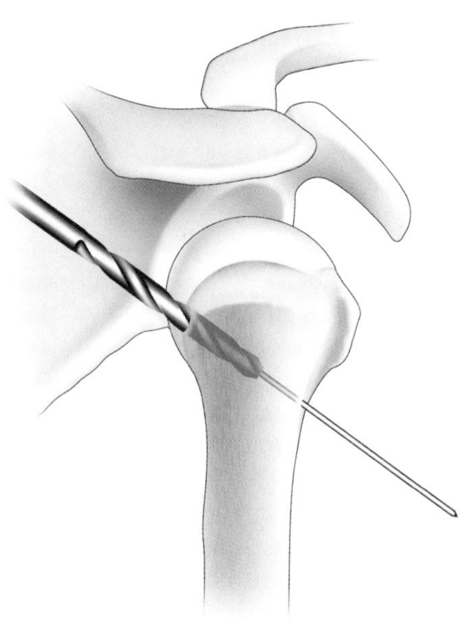

Fig. 5 – The KWire (with a guide) crossing the humeral head, to the bicipital groove.

The entry point is identified and 20 mm Kirshner wire is drilled at 45° angle to the humeral head aiming toward the bicipital groove anteriorly. It crosses the humeral head from posterior and superior to anterior and inferior (Fig. 5). A 6 mm tunnel is made around the KWire. The passage of the tendon into the tunnel remains technically delicate under arthroscopy because of "acute" angle that the tendon takes. We advise to put a second traction suture at the junction muscle/tendon to facilitate this passage, and in parallel to slacken traction in the axis of the arm to be able to mobilize it more easily. The tension on the pedicle is controlled by two sutures placed 4 cm apart on the muscle belly. A titanium or resorbable interference screw is then introduced, diameter 8 mm (two sizes bigger drill) and length 23 mm (Fig. 6), to fix the tendon.

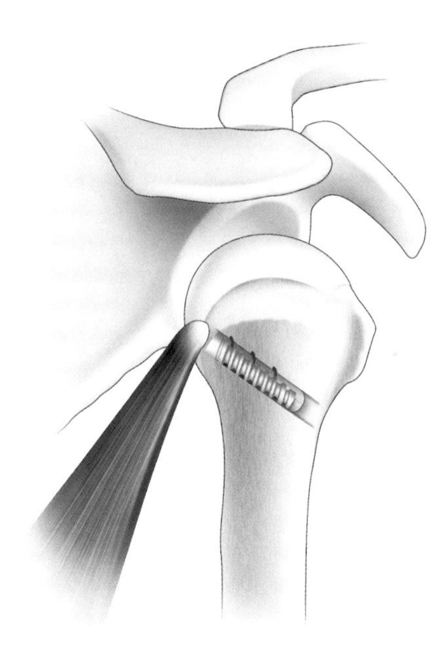

Fig. 6 – Massive and posterosuperior cuff tear. LD transfer with IFS by arthroscopic procedure.

Technique with closed tunnel

This technique was first introduced by Philippe Valenti. The advantage is that the surgeon is free from the way out. Drill is directly realized into the humeral head, where bone is always good. With a biotenodesis 8 mm screw, the tendon is introduced and fixed into the hole. An additional anchor can be used laterally to the tunnel to prevent a winds wiper effect.

Reverse IFS: TLS technique

In case of grossly osteoporotic humeral head, we feel IFS may not be a strong fixation. We advocate the TLS technic, developed for ACL reconstruction by Xavier Cassard et al. Steps are exactly the same, but this technic is a little more demanding. After drilling, one has to look at the KWire way out at the bicipital groove, to control the distal to proximal fixation by TLS screw. This screw is introduced with the KWire guide, between the two tapes. Fixation is cortical anteriorly around the bstrong bicipital groove stronger than in the direct IFS technique, with 100% tendon-bone fixation. The biomechanical superiority has been proved.

Technique with classic anchors (Milliet)

Milliet (12) in 2007 introduced arthroscopic technique of LDT fixation. He proposed a beach chair position, but dissection of LD seems more difficult. Similar to our IFS technique, the interval underneath the deltoid and posterior to the teres minor is developed by blunt dissection to create a subdeltoid tunnel.

No. 2 fiberwire suture is used to pull the tendon and maintain tension. Then, three BioCorkscrew anchors are used in a diamond double-row pattern to secure the LDT into place onto the footprint of the greater tuberosity. The no. 2 fiberwire sutures are then secured to the subscapularis arthroscopically closing the rotator interval. It seems to us more demanding and more time consuming and cumbersome perform. In case of bad bone quality, classics anchors may not be enough strong.

References

1. Warner JJ (2001) Management of massive irreparable rotator cuff tears: the role of tendon transfer. J Shoulder Elbow Surg; 10(6): 514-521
2. Gerber C, Vinh TS, Hertel R, Hess CW (1988) Latissimus dorsi transfer for the treatment of massive tears of the rotator cuff. A preliminary report. Clin Orthop; 232: 51-61
3. Phipps GJ, Hoffer MM (1995)Latissimus dorsi and teres major transfer to rotator cuff for Erb's palsy. J Shoulder Elbow Surg; 4(2): 124-129
4. Gerber C (1992) Latissimus dorsi transfer for the treatment of irreparable tears of the rotator cuff. Clin Orthop; 275: 152-160

5. Miniaci A, Mcleod M (1999) Transfer of the latissimus dorsi muscle after failed repair of a massive tear of the rotator cuff. A two to five-year review. J Bone Joint Surg Am; 81(8): 1120-1127
6. Irlenbusch U, Bracht M, Gansen HK, Lorenz U, Thiel J (2008) Latissimus dorsi transfer for irreparable rotator cuff tears: a longitudinal study. J Shoulder Elbow Surg; 17(4): 527-34
7. Irlenbusch U, Bensdorf M, Gansen HK, Lorenz U (2003) Latissimus dorsi transfer in case of irreparable rotator cuff tear: a comparative analysis of primary and failed rotator cuff surgery, in dependence of deficiency grade and additional lesions. Z Orthop Ihre Grenzgeb; 141(6): 650-656
8. Aldrige JM, Atkinson TS, Mallon WJ (2004) Combined pectoralis major and latissimus dorsi tendon transfer for massive rotator cuff deficiency. J Shoulder Elbow Surg; 13(6): 621-629
9. Degreef I, Debeer P, Van Herck B, Van Den Eeden E, Peers K, De Smet L (2005) Treatment of irreparable rotator cuff tears by latissimus dorsi muscle transfer. Acta Orthop Belg; 71(6): 667-671
10. Iannotti JP, Hennigan S, Herzog R, Kella S, Kelley M, Leggin B, Williams GR (2006) Latissimus dorsi tendon transfer for irreparable posterosuperior rotator cuff tears. Factors affecting outcome. J Bone Joint Surg Am; 88(2): 342-348
11. Boileau P, Krishnan S, Coste JS, Walch G (2001) Arthroscopic biceps tenodesis: a new technic using interference screw. Tech Shoulder Elbow Surg; 2(3): 153-165
12. Milliet PJ, Yen Y-M, Huang MJ (2008) Arthroscopically assisted latissimus dorsi transfer for irreparable rotator cuff tears. Tech Shoulder Elbow Surg; 9(2): 76-79

Teres major flap: surgical anatomy, technique of harvesting, methods of fixation, postoperative management

P. Mansat, A. Dotziz, Y. Bellumore, M. Mansat

Introduction

Massive rotator cuff ruptures in patients younger than 65 years represent a therapeutic challenge. Loss of function of the infraspinatus leads to loss of active external rotation and anterior elevation, and upward migration of the humeral head. Combined transfer of latissimus dorsi and teres major has been used since many years to treat sequellae of obstetrical plexus palsy with loss of active external rotation (1-3). Gerber et al., in 1988, first described the use of latissimus dorsi muscle transfer to treat massive rotator cuff tear (4). In 1993, Combes and Mansat (5) performed an anatomical study and showed that the teres major had a vascular and nervous autonomy, and that the biometry of the muscle and the length of its pedicle allowed for transfer of its tendon to the humeral head. Later, other anatomical studies have confirmed these results (6-8). Celli et al. (9) published the first clinical series in 1998 with encouraging results. More recently, some authors have studied the combined transfer of the latissimus dorsi and teres major to treat massive rotator cuff tears involving mainly the supraspinatus and infraspinatus tendons (8). The goal of the different transfer was to recover an external rotation of the shoulder and to obtain a depressor effect on the humeral head to compensate the absence of the supraspinatus and infraspinatus muscles.

Anatomy of the teres major muscle

Descriptive anatomy

The teres major is a thick but somewhat flattened muscle, which arises from the oval area on the dorsal surface of the inferior angle of the scapula, and from the fibrous septa interposed between the muscle and the teres minor and infraspinatus; the fibers are directed upward and lateralward, and end in a flat tendon, about 5 cm long, which is inserted into the crest of the lesser tubercle of the humerus. The tendon, at its insertion, lies behind that of the latissimus dorsi, from which it is separated by a bursa, the two tendons being, however, united along their lower borders for a short distance estimated at 3.0 cm for Wang et al. (6). The teres major tendon is partially covered posteriorly by muscle fibers that attached directly to the periosteum of the humerus; the tendinous portion was on the anterior surface. The clinical significance of this partial concealment is that the tendon may be longer than is readily apparent (6) (Fig. 1).

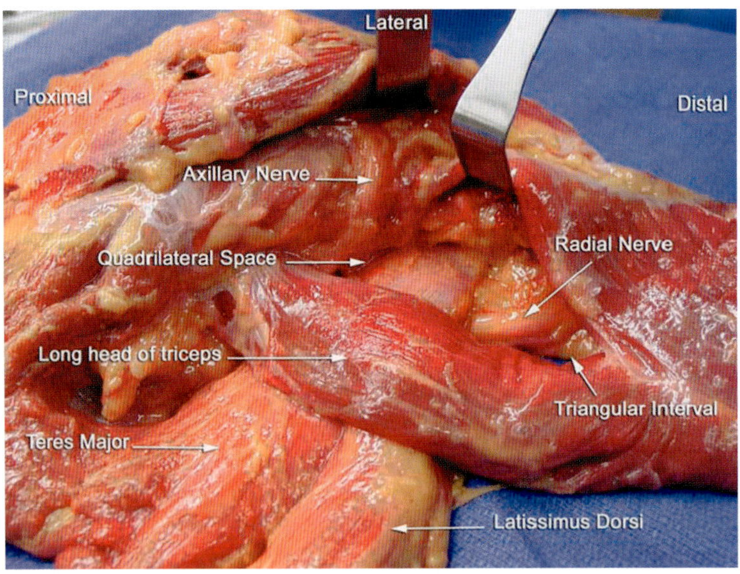

Fig. 1 – Anatomical view of the muscular and neurological structures around the teres major muscle at the posterior aspect of the shoulder. From Ref. (13) (Copyright © 2007, The Journal of Bone and Joint Surgery, Inc.).

Dimensions of the teres major

In their anatomical study Combes and Mansat (5) found that the average muscle length averaged 11.7 cm (±0.9). The terminal tendon is large with a trapezoidal shape with an average of 3.3 cm (±0.8 mm) length at its humeral insertion. The average distance between the muscle insertion on the scapula and the greater tubercle averaged 18.5 cm (±5.7 mm). The average rotation arc of the teres major muscle after it has been dissected to reach the humeral head was of 27.3° (±2.1°). For Wang et al. (6) the mean tendon length was 2.0 cm and the mean muscle length was 11.8 cm. For Pearle et al. (8) the average width of the teres major tendon at its insertion site was 4.0 cm (3.3-5), and the average length was 3.9 cm (3.3-4.6).

Vascular supply

The vascular supply of the teres major muscle derived from the circumflex scapular artery, a branch of the subscapular artery. The teres major appeared to have a predominant artery. In Combes and Mansat' studies (5), the predominant artery was a branch of the subscapular artery in 2/3 of the cases. However, vascular supply came also from one or more arteries from the periscapular arterial circle. It could be classified as Mathes type II (one predominant artery and accessories arteries) (10). In Wang et al.'s study (6), 3 specimens out of 11 had Mathes type I circulation, arising from the circumflex scapular artery and one specimen had Mathes type IV circulation, arising directly from the subscapular artery. In Wang et al.'s studies (6), the dominant vascular pedicle entered the anterosuperior edge of the muscle at an average of 4.1 cm (range 2.2-6.5 cm) from the superior scapular origin of the muscle. The secondary pedicles also arose from the circumflex scapular artery and entered the muscle belly approximately 0.5 cm (range 0.2-1.0 cm) from the muscle origin. For Combes and Mansat (5), the length of the artery of the teres major from its origin was 35 mm (23-41 mm) with a cross-section diameter of 1-2 mm.

Nerve supply

The nerve to the teres major, the lower subscapular nerve, arose consistently from the posterior cord of the brachial plexus and entered, with the artery, the anterosuperior edge of the muscle at approximately 4.1 cm (range 2.0-6.2 cm) from the scapular origin (6). The teres major was entered by a dominant neurovascular pedicle through its anterosuperior surface. The relation of the entry point of the main neurovascular bundle to the total length of the teres major was relatively constant. If the landmarks of the muscle's origin (inferior border of the scapula) and insertion (border of the humerus) were considered, the pedicle entered the muscle at approximately the medial 30% of the muscle (range 15-50%).

Study of the tension of the vascular-nervous pedicle after teres major transfer

In Combes and Mansat's study (5), the transfer of the teres major muscle has always been possible because of the pedicle length. The tendon could reach easily the greater tuberosity after being passed under the deltoid muscle. Even in maximal abduction there was no excessive traction on the pedicle.

Knowledge of the location of the neurovascular pedicle insertions into the teres major muscle allows axial dissection of the muscle off the latissimus dorsi muscle and thus minimizes the chance of nerve or vessel injury. Awareness of the proximity of the posterior branch of the axillary nerve to the transferred tendon beneath the posterior deltoid allows for safer passage of the tendons (Fig. 2).

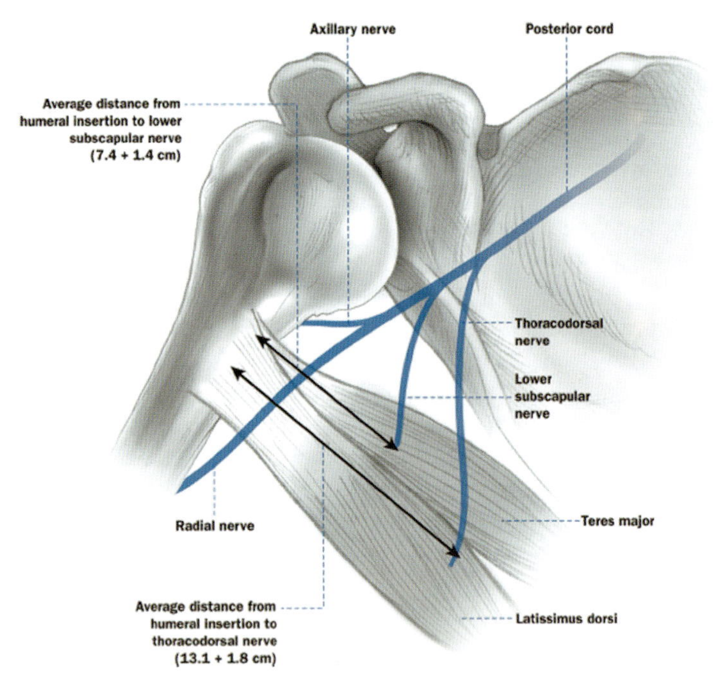

Fig. 2 – Relationships between the radial and axillary nerves from the tendons of the latissimus dorsi and teres major. From Ref. (8) (Copyright © 2006, The Journal of Bone and Joint Surgery, Inc.).

Biomechanics of teres major flap

In 2004, Magermans et al. (11) have shown on a biomechanical musculoskeletal model that after transfer of the teres major on the supraspinatus and/or infraspinatus or teres minor tendons, its moment arm changes from a retroflexor to an anteflexor. The moment arm of the teres major is 1.7 cm when attached to the infraspinatus, 0.7 cm when attached to the teres minor, 2.0 cm when attached to the supraspinatus, and 1.2 cm when attached to the subscapularis. An external rotation function is obtained when transferred to supraspinatus and in particular when transferred to the infraspinatus insertion. The moment arm after transfer to the subscapularis and teres minor insertions remains positive; in other words, the muscle remains an internal rotator. Due to the difference in moment arm, the teres major is required to generate 10 N less force when transferred to the infraspinatus insertion than when transferred to the supraspinatus insertion. On the basis of mechanical parameters such as moment arms, muscle length, and force, it can be concluded that a tendon transfer of the teres major to the supraspinatus insertion will produce the best functional outcome in the treatment of massive rotator cuff tears.

In 2006, de Groot et al. (12) have shown that teres major activation adapts to both pathological and postsurgery conditions: the normal activation during adduction changes into activation during forward flexion or abduction. Glenohumeral stabilization seems to be the explanation for postsurgery teres major transfer success. Indeed, the pathological absence of supraspinatus and infraspinatus forces during forward flexion result in increased upward glenohumeral instability. The superior translations are compensated for by teres major activity during forward flexion. This translation-'force' function conflicts with the adduction-generating rotation-'torque' function. This may explain the pain-induced reduction of arm elevation in these patients. Musculotendinous transfer solves the force-torque conflict by changing the moment arm of the teres major from adduction to abduction. Teres major can now both compensate for the loss of supraspinatus and infraspinatus forces needed for glenohumeral stabilization and contribute to forward flexion of the arm.

Surgical technique

Anesthesia

The surgery is performed under general anesthesia with interscalenic block to control pain level postoperatively.

Installation

The patient is positioned in the lateral decubitus position and stabilized with a sandbag, and the entire limb and hemithorax are draped free in the sterile field. The contour of the scapula is drawn including the scapula spine as well as the posterior axillary line (Fig. 3).

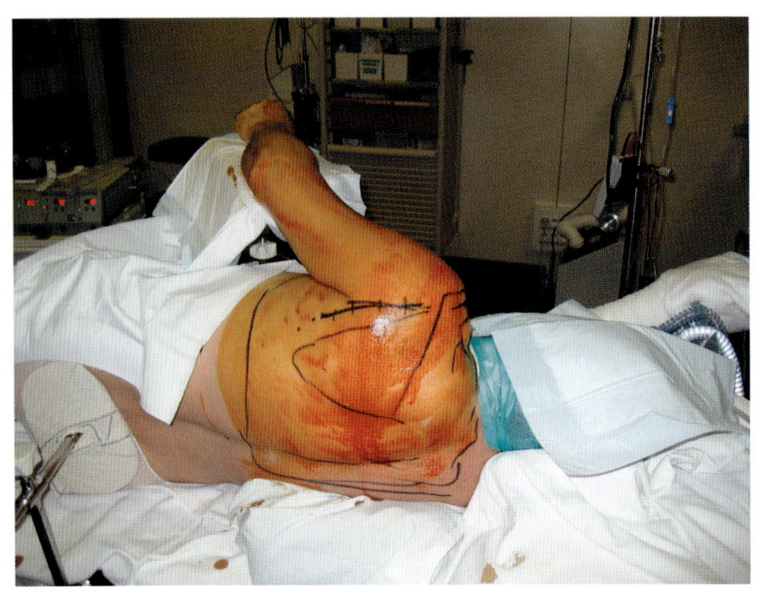

Fig. 3 – Patient installation and bony landmarks.

Superior incision

A two-incision approach is utilized. First, the rotator cuff is approached through a superior incision. The anterior fascial raphe of the deltoid is identified and split, with care taken not to extend the split more than 5 cm distal to the acromion to avoid injury to the axial nerve. The anterior portion of the deltoid is released from the acromion. An acromioplasty is systematically performed. The rotator cuff is inspected, and an attempt is made to mobilize a sufficient amount of retracted rotator cuff tissue to perform a tension-free primary repair. Lysis of adhesions, resection of the coracohumeral ligament, and a capsular release may be necessary to free the retracted tendon tissue adequately. If it is determined that a primary repair cannot be performed, then the teres major transfer is carried out.

Posterior incision

Attention is then turned to the posterior aspect of the shoulder. The skin incision is posterior of 7-10 cm length from 2 cm under the spine of the scapula vertically to reach the posterior axillary line.

Teres major harvesting

The superficial layers are dissected until the aponeurosis of the infraspinatus is reached. The aponeurosis is then open just on the teres major and latissimus dorsi muscle. The two muscles are then separated gently from the scapula border to their tendinous termination. It is not necessary to dissect the pedicle of the teres major. The arm is positioned in internal rotation to slacken the teres major muscle and to bring its humeral insertion more superficial. With this maneuver, an average of 1.9 cm (range 1.5-2.4 cm) of additional teres major tendon tissue can be visualized as compared with that seen in neutral rotation (13) (Fig. 4). The long head of the triceps is retracted. The tendon is then desinserted from the bone. Caution is observed in order not to damage the tendon of the latissimus dorsi muscle. The free tendon is then released (Fig. 5). The teres major tendon is then tagged with heavy number 5 braided sutures in a Krakow pattern and is freely mobilized in preparation to transfer. While traction is applied to the tagging sutures, the teres major tendon and its muscle bellies are dissected free from the latissimus dorsi. This axial dissection is carried out until the tendon has enough excursion to reach the posterolateral border of the acromion. At the inferior border of the teres major tendon, which extends distal to the latissimus dorsi tendon, the radial nerve is an average of 2.3 cm medial to the humerus. The axillary nerve lies at an average of 1.4 cm (range 0.8-2.0 cm) proximal to the upper edge of the teres major, which extends superior to the latissimus dorsi tendon at this level (8, 13).

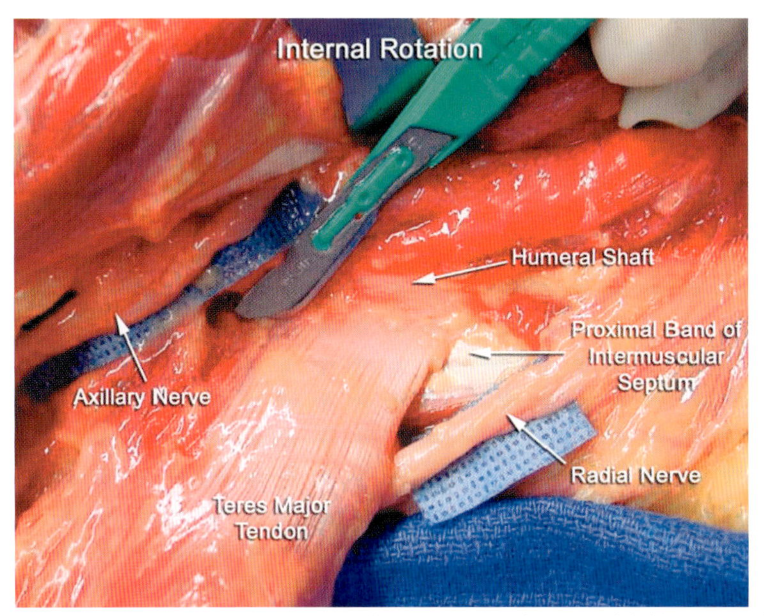

Fig. 4 – Maximum internal rotation delivers the tendons into the surgical field. From Ref. (13) (Copyright © 2007, The Journal of Bone and Joint Surgery, Inc.).

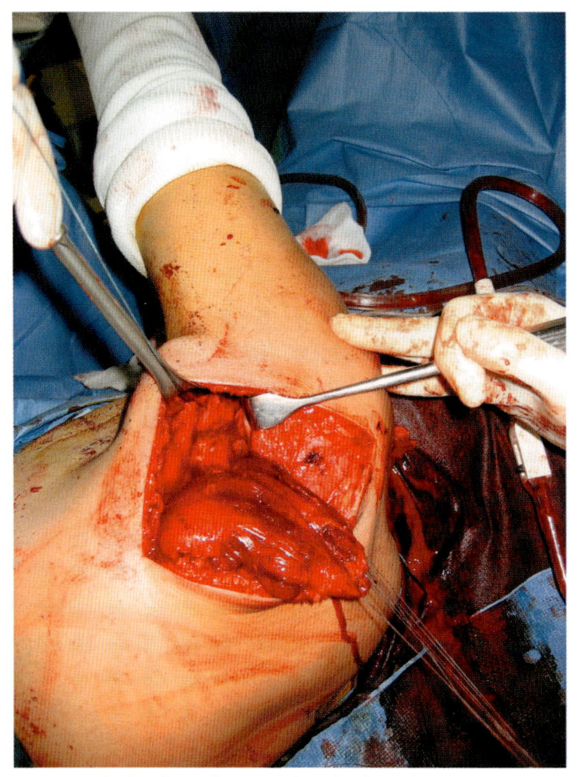

Fig. 5 – Teres major muscle has been harvested and released.

Transfer of the teres major

When the tendons are fully mobilized, preparation is made for tunneling the musculotendinous units under the posterior portion of the deltoid and superficial to the infraspinatus and teres minor. The plane between the posterior part of the deltoid and the rotator cuff muscles is identified, and the posterior part of the deltoid is gently retracted laterally. A clamp is guided through the anterior incision, under the deltoid and into the subacromial space, and out through the posterior incision, creating a tunnel for tendon passage. During this last step, care is taken not to injure the posterior branch of the axillary nerve that lies in the deep fascia of the deltoid. The teres major is pull until the tendon reaches the humeral head (Fig. 6). Freedom of the muscle must be controlled all along its way when moving the arm. The tendon is then sutured to the remnant of the rotator cuff and to the greater tuberosity through transosseous bone sutures or suture anchors. The remnant of the native rotator cuff is repaired in a side-to-side manner to the transferred tendons (Fig. 7). Mobilization of the shoulder in all planes allows the surgeon to evaluate the adequate tension of the transfer.

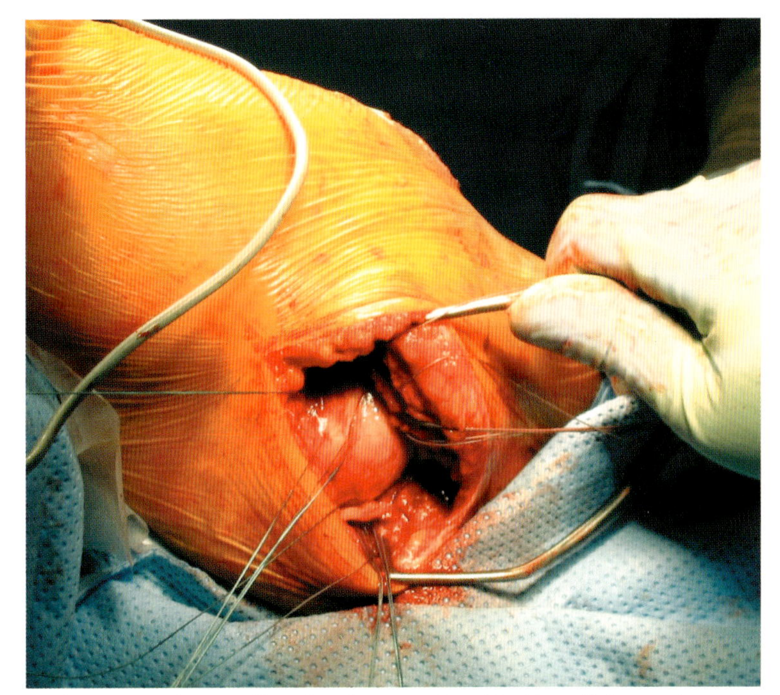

Fig. 6 – The teres major is pull under the posterior deltoid until the tendon reaches the humeral head.

Closure

The anterior deltoid is sutured to the median deltoid and to the acromion. Both incisions are closed in two layers on a suction drain.

Postoperative

The patient is placed in an abduction splint for 6 weeks. Passive motion starts after 2 weeks with pendulum exercises allowed. Active-assist motion is started at 6 weeks with supine forward elevation and rotation movements. Care is taken to reestablish adequate glenohumeral and scapulothoracic rhythms. At 12 weeks postoperatively, the patient starts active supine range-of-motion exercises and progresses with active motion and strengthening.

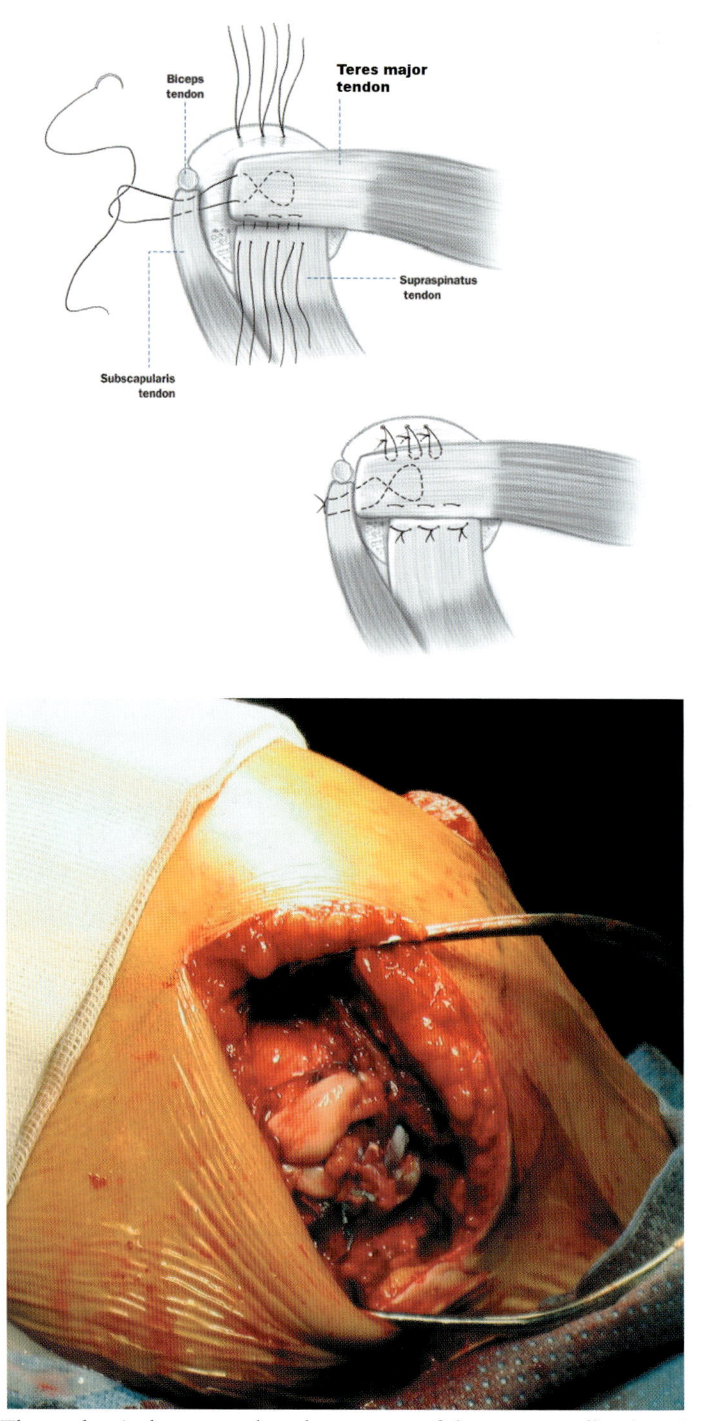

Fig. 7 – The tendon is then sutured to the remnant of the rotator cuff and to the greater tuberosity through transosseous bone sutures or suture anchors.

Clinical experience

Patients

Between 1992 and 2004, a teres major muscle transfer was performed on 12 patients with non-reparable massive rotator cuff tears. There were 2 women and 10 men, of 49 years of age on average. The dominant side was involved in 8. In nine cases, the patients were already operated for a cuff rupture.

Preoperative evaluation was performed with a clinical examination and the Constant score. Standard radiographs (AP view in three rotations and Neer view) and MRI or arthro-CT were also performed. A combined supraspinatus and infraspinatus tears was observed in nine patients, but in three only an isolated infraspinatus lesion was found. In all cases, the fatty degeneration index was greater than 2. The tear was posttraumatic in six cases and degenerative in six (Table I).

In eight cases, an isolated teres major muscle transfer was performed, but in four cases a combined teres major/latissimus dorsi transfer was preferred.

Postoperative evaluation was performed clinically with the Constant score and radiographically with standard radiographs of the shoulder. An MRI was performed in five, as well as an EMG study.

Table I – Characteristics of patients included in the study.

Patient	*Age (years)*	*Tear*	*Transfer*	*F/u (year)*
1	42	Supra + infra (traumatic)	TM	13
2	70	Supra + infra (degenerative)	TM+LD	Lost F/u
3	38	Supra + infra (traumatic)	TM	12
4	44	Supra + infra (traumatic)	TM	12
5	45	Supra + infra (degenerative)	TM	11
6	64	Supra + infra (degenerative)	TM+LD	9
7	44	Supra + infra (traumatic)	TM+LD	5
8	51	Supra + infra (degenerative)	TM+LD	5
9	47	Infra (traumatic)	TM	2
10	54	Infra (degenerative)	TM	2
11	49	Infra (degenerative)	TM	1
12	41	Supra + infra (traumatic)	TM	1

Supra, supraspinatus tendon; infra, infraspinatus tendon; TM, teres major; LD, latissimus dorsi.

Results

Follow-up

One patient was lost for follow-up. Eleven patients could be reviewed at 6 years average follow-up (1-13 years).

Clinical evaluation

The Constant score improved for a mean of 38 points preoperatively to 60 points postoperatively with an average gain of 22 points. Pain score improved significantly with an average gain of 6.22 points postoperatively. Range of motion improved mainly in anterior elevation, seven patients reaching more than 90° elevation. External rotation improved slightly with an average gain of 12.7° (Table II).

Table II – Preoperative and postoperative evaluation of the Constant score.

Patient	*Constant pre-op (points)*	*Constant post-op (points)*	*Gain (points)*
1	35	37	+2
3	31	52	+21
4	46	60	+14
5	34	59	+25
6	24	39	+15
7	41	55	+14
8	39.5	65	+25.5
9	47	85	+38
10	45	72	+27
11	47	80	+33
12	36	61	+25

Radiographic evaluation

On radiographic evaluation, the humeral head stayed upward migrated in all cases in neutral position but tended to be recentered at 90° abduction. Shoulder centered preoperatively stayed centered postoperatively. Sign of osteoarthritis appeared between 6 and 9 years after the transfer procedure.

Electromyographic and MRI evaluation

EMG studies of the teres major performed in five patients showed activation of the muscle in all cases while the patient tending to elevate their arm. MRI in the same group of patients showed no degenerative evolution of the teres major with an index at 0 at the last follow-up (Fig. 8).

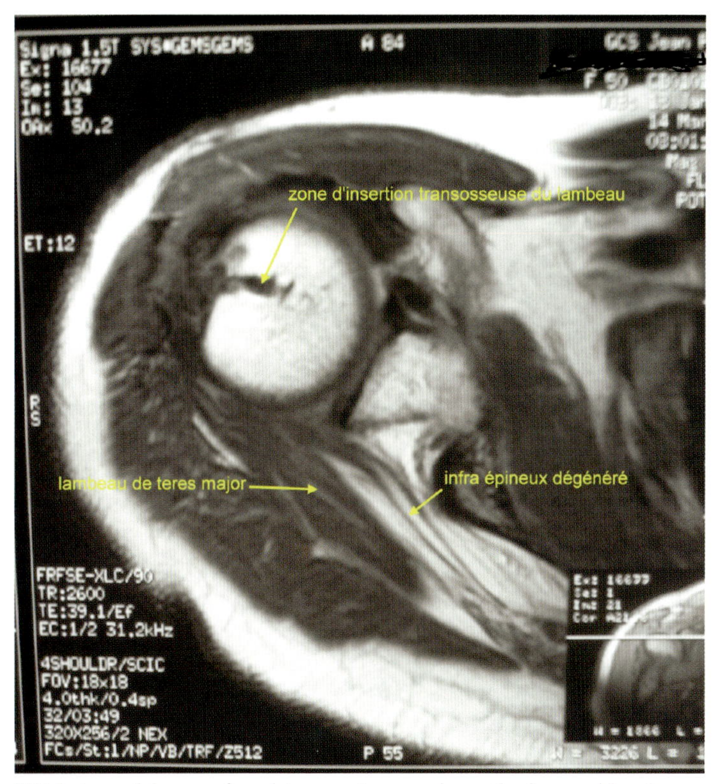

Fig. 8 – MRI view of the transferred teres major muscle on the humeral head.

Complication

There was one complication. A patient with a massive rotator cuff tear with upward migration of the humeral head and no more acromio-humeral space had a quick degradation of the muscle transfer. The transfer did not depress the humeral head and the muscle transfer deteriorated with time rubbing on the acromion. A shoulder arthroplasty was performed 6 years after the transfer procedure.

Prognosis factors

Negative prognosis factors were: previous surgery, anterior extension of the cuff tear with involvement of the subscapularis tendon, and importance of the preoperative functional deficit. Positive prognosis factors were: isolated involvement of the infraspinatus tendon, preoperative active external rotation with an active teres minor muscle, and preservation of the subscapularis anteriorly. Patients with positive prognosis factors had a gain of 30 points on average of the Constant score.

Discussion

In shoulder abduction, the integrity of the posterior cuff, not only of the supraspinatus, is essential to maintain the balance between the force couples on the vertical and horizontal planes, thus ensuring the permanent static and dynamic recentering of the humeral head (9). To obtain a full elevation, external rotation is needed. During anteflexion and abduction approximately 50° of humeral external rotation was used. The main cause for not meeting the constraints is that in the healthy situation there are only a few muscles (infraspinatus, teres minor, and a small part of the supraspinatus) that are able to produce an external rotation moment around the glenohumeral joint (11).

In 1993, Combes and Mansat (5) have shown through an anatomical study that the teres major had morphologic characteristics and an autonomous neurovascular pedicle that allowed using it as a transfer. Other anatomical studies have later confirmed these results (6-8).

Biomechanical studies have then shown that the two main functions of the rotator cuff muscles, stabilizing the glenohumeral joint and aiding the prime movers of the humerus, can be completely fulfilled by the teres major (11). These studies outlined that after transfer the change of moment arms of the teres major turns the muscle into an external rotator and elevator of the humerus during anteflexion and abduction.

Celli et al. (9) have first published a clinical series of teres major muscle transfer to treat irreparable rotor cuff tears involving the infraspinatus tendon. Patients had no major degenerative osteoarticular alteration, passive external rotation was still present, and the supraspinatus was still functional or its function could be restored through a direct reconstruction or transfer. Six patients have been operated with this procedure. At 14 months average follow-up, Constant score improved from 40 to 62 points postoperatively. Active external rotation recovered 35° in abduction to 90° and 24° in adduction. More recently, Celli et al. (14) have updated these results and 20 patients of 61 years average age, operated with a teres major muscle transfer, were reviewed with 36 months average follow-up (14-65). All patients had tears of supraspinatus and infraspinatus tendon with stages 3-4 fatty degeneration of the muscles. The mean Constant score improved from 31.6 to 66.1 points. Pain level decreased significantly with a postoperative score of 14.2 points out of 15 points. Active anterior elevation increased from 92° to 147°, and external rotation from 7° to 26.5°. Force increased slightly from a mean value of 1 kg preoperatively to

1.5 kg postoperatively. MRI evaluation showed one case of partial tendinous disinsertion of the transfer. No case of teres major atrophy was found. EMG analysis showed the functional activity of the transfer during active movements of abduction and external rotation.

From our experience and the series published in the literature, our indications of teres major muscle transfer have been focused. Indications are limited to patients under 55 years of age, who well understand the surgical procedure and the rehabilitation program. Ideal indication concerns isolated tendon tear of the infraspinatus tendon or in association with the posterior part of the supraspinatus tendon. The anterior part of the supraspinatus tendon and the subscapularis tendon must be intact. In case of massive cuff tear involving all the supraspinatus tendon up to the upper part of the subscapularis tendon and the infraspinatus tendon, a combined transfer of the teres major and the latissimus dorsi muscles must be preferred. Celli et al. (9) have written that the transfer of the teres major muscle seems logical because of the following:

- it is physiologically more like the infraspinatus because it is a scapulohumeral muscle;
- it can be transferred into the infraspinatus fossa and its orientation superimposed on the infraspinatus;
- its tendon is long enough to be inserted into the greater tuberosity;
- the surgical operation does not present major technical difficulties.

The disadvantages are as follows:

- it can be difficult to establish the correct tension in the transfer into the greater tuberosity; tension must be determined by assessing the presence of satisfactory internal rotators and the passive motion in internal and external rotation to prevent the loss of internal rotation;
- the transfer of the teres major cannot completely replace supraspinatus function, especially regarding the superioinferior and anteroposterior plane stability that is essential for a dynamic recentering of the humeral head;
- the insertion on the greater tuberosity must be localized in the infraspinatus seat.

References

1. L'Episcopo JB (1934) Tendon transplantation in obstetrical paralysis. Am J Surg; 25: 122
2. Hoffer MM, Wickender R, Roper B (1978) Brachial plexus birth palsies. Results of tendon transfers to the rotator cuff. J Bone Joint Surg Am; 60: 691-695
3. Zancolli EA, Zancolli ER Jr (1988) Palliative surgical procedure for sequelae of obstetrical palsy. Hand Clin; 4: 643-648
4. Gerber C, Vinh TS, Hertel R, Hess CW (1988) Latissimus dorsi transfer for the treatment of massive tears of the rotator cuff. Clin Orthop; 232: 51-61

5. Combes JM, Mansat M (1993) Lambeau du muscle grand rond dans les ruptures massives de la coiffe des rotateurs. Etude expérimentale. In: «L'Epaule» de Bonnel F, Blotman F, Mansat M, Editeurs. Paris: Springer-Verlag France: 318-330
6. Wang A, Strauch R, Flatow E (1999) The Teres Major muscle: an anatomic study of its use as a tendon transfer. J Shoulder Elbow Surg; 8: 334-338
7. Schoierer O, Herzberg G, Berthonnaud E, Dimnet J, Aswad R, Morin A (2001) Anatomical basis of Latissimus dorsi and Teres major transfers in rotator cuff tear surgery with particular reference to the neurovascular pedicles. Surg Radiol Anat; 23: 75-80
8. Pearle AD, Kelly BT, Voos JE, Chehab EL, Warren RF (2006) Surgical technique and anatomic study of Latissimus Dorsi and Teres Major transfers. J Bone Joint Surg Am; 88: 1524-1531
9. Celli L, Rovesta C, Marongiu MC, Manzieri S (1998) Transplantation of teres major muscle for infraspinatus muscle in irreparable rotator cuff tears. J Shoulder Elbow Surg; 7: 485-490
10. Mathes SJ, Nahai F (1981) Classification of the vascular anatomy of muscles experimental and clinical correlations. Plast Reconstr Surg; 67: 177-187
11. Magermans DJ, Chadwick EKJ, Veeger HEJ, van der Helm FCT, PM Rozing (2004) Biomechanical analysis of tendon transfers for massive rotator cuff tears. Clin Biomech; 19: 350-357
12. de Groot JH, van de Sande MAJ, Meskers CGM, Rozing PM (2006) Pathological Teres Major activation in patients with massive rotator cuff tears alters with pain relief and/or salvage surgery transfer. Clin Biomech; 21: S27-S32
13. Pearle AD, Voos JE, Kelly BT, Chehab EL, Warren RF (2007) Surgical technique and anatomic study of Latissimus Dorsi and Teres Major transfers. Surgical technique. J Bone Joint Surg Am; 89: 284-296
14. Celli A, Maronqiu MC, Rovesta C, Celli L (2005) Transplant of the teres major in the treatment of irreparable injuries of the rotator cuff (long-term analysis of results). Chir Organi Mov; 90: 121-132

Deltoid flap for irreparable rotator cuff tear: indications, technique and results

D. Katz, H. Thomazeau, J.E. Gedouin, M. Colmar

Introduction

Initially described by Takagishi (1) the deltoid flap has been widely used since the modification of the original technique by two French surgeons Apoil and Augereau (2).

The original Japanese technique consisted of taking the anterior and lateral part of the deltoid muscle while the French team described the elevation of only the anterior acromial part of the muscle. This lessens the morbidity of the sample and allows an easier closure of the donor site.

Even today the irreparable cuff tear in young patients remains a problem and subject to discussions. The choice goes from a simple arthroscopic debridement without repair, a full transposition of the tendinomuscular structure, a tendon transfer such as latissimus dorsi, a prosthetic tendon (3).

The deltoid flap is a local flap elevated using the same incision than a classic direct suture technique. This allows a late peroperative decision.

The authors had previously reported a good pain relief obtained but the final strength in this preliminary report was low and some patients with an intact preoperative active elevation had lost some mobility (4).

A clinical and radiological evaluation seemed to be accurate with a long-term follow-up (5).

Indications and contraindications

The deltoid flap should be considered as an alternative solution in front of a big irreparable rotator cuff tear using the conventional techniques of suturing. It should be reserved to patients in good health, less than 65 years with irretractable pain after medical treatment and rehabilitation attempts for more than 6 months.

However, our recurrent and long-term review of patients has shown that the deltoid flap must not be used in cases of normal preoperative anterior active elevation (see below). Moreover, the patient must be warned not to expect a good final strength as it can be less than half of the normal side. This can be a problem in heavy workers who are not yet retired. Many studies have shown that a preoperative big loss of strength will not be corrected by the flap, and this precludes a return to heavy work in more than half of the cases.

Some results have shown that the deltoid flap is not a good indication in anterior tears involving the subscapularis tendon. Of course the deltoid muscle must be functional and paralysis of the axillary nerve is a contraindication.

Preoperative planning

The preoperative planning includes the complete clinical evaluation of the active and passive motion, and the elements of the Constant score such as quantified pain, strength, and activities of daily leaving.

It needs also a good imaging:

- The classical four normal X-rays in AP view (rotation 0°, lateral and medial rotation, and Lamy sagittal radiograph). We advise also to do a good measurement of the subacromial space with a double oblique view.
- MRI, arthro-MRI, or arthroscan are the good way of appreciation of the soft tissues lesions: number of tendons involved, degree of retraction, and quality of the muscles.

Surgical technique

The patient is placed in a beach chair position. The approach is superior with two variations:

- A superior and anterior approach, from the acromio-clavicular joint following the anterior edge of the anterior acromial part of the deltoid muscle. A fatty line is often seen between the clavicular and the acromial part of the deltoid muscle which makes the dissection of the future anterior edge of the flap easier (Fig. 1).
- The classic superior approach, following the bony anterior edge of the acromion. We advise to make the incision half a centimeter on the bone, in order to detach a periosteal flap in continuity with the acromio-coracoid ligament (6) (Fig. 2). This reinforces the future posterior edge of the deltoid flap. The splitting of the muscle starts at the anterolateral corner of the acromion for 3-4 cm long. A small trick is useful to avoid any risk for

the axillary nerve during the splitting of the muscle (Fig. 3). As soon as the subacromial space is open, it is possible to introduce a finger into the subacromial bursa. The split must not go under the bottom of the bursa.

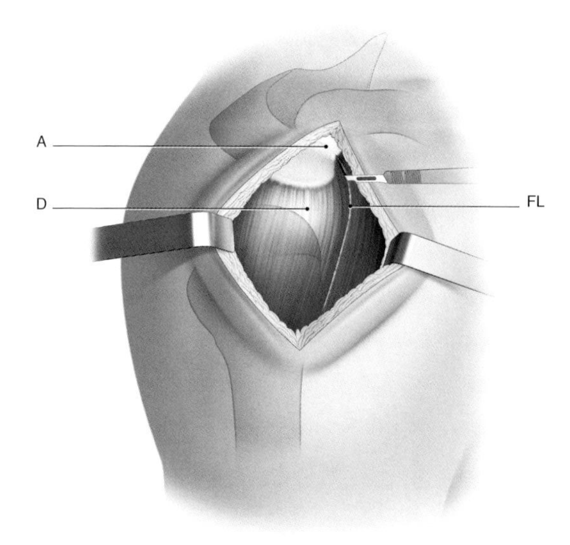

Fig. 1 – Anterolateral approach.
A: Acromion; D: Deltoid muscle; FL: Fatty line.

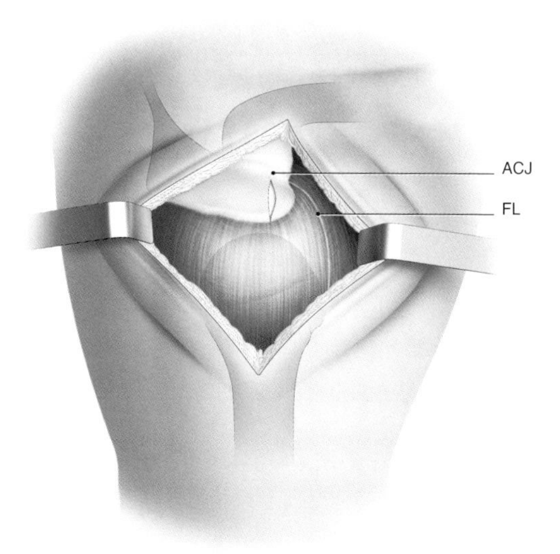

Fig. 2 – Detachment of the periosteal flap in continuity with the acromio-coracoid ligament.
ACJ: Acromioclavicular joint; FL: Fatty line.

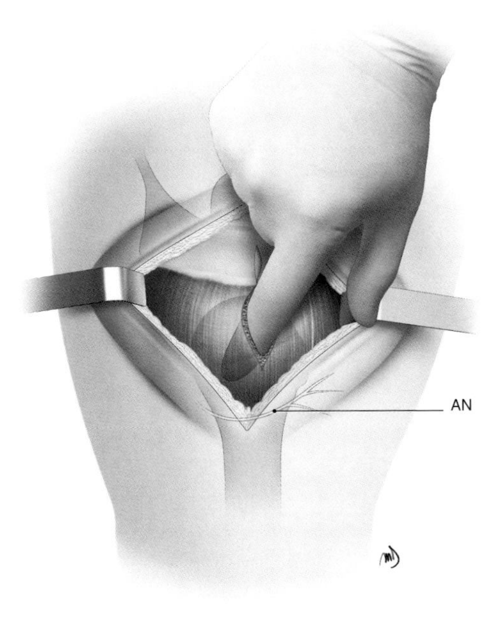

Fig. 3 – Discision between the anterior and the middle fibres of the deltoid.
AN: Axillary nerve.

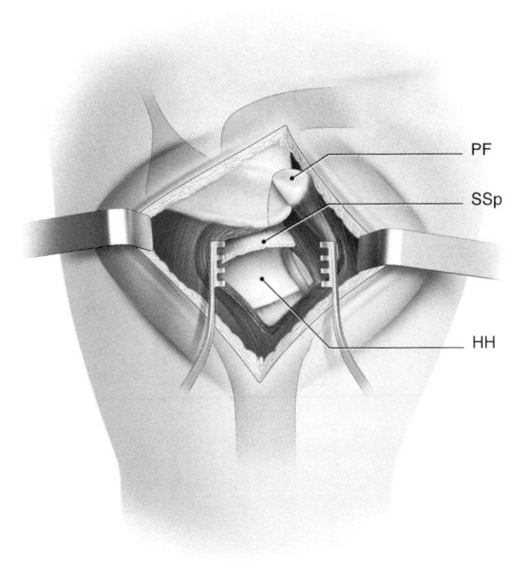

Fig. 4 – Supraspinatus is retracted and not repairable.
PF: Periosteal flap; SSp: Supraspinatus; HH: Humeral head.

The decision between those two approaches is decided preoperatively depending on the size of the tear. If the rupture is mainly posterior (it is often the case when choosing a deltoid flap) the classic superior approach is chosen. If the tear has an anterior extension the anterosuperior approach can be chosen giving a good view to the anterior edge of the tear.

The operation starts with a good exposition of the lesions (Fig. 4). The deltoid flap is often chosen at this moment (50% of the cases in our series (5)), in front of an irreparable tear by the classical techniques of repair. An acromioplasty is done; an acromio-clavicular plasty is realized in case of arthritis, often useful to enhance the vision of the medial edge of the tear. The flap must be able to cover the defect and sutured in place without tension even with the elbow on body.

If the flap is decided then starts its release. We have already described the search of the fatty line between the clavicular and the acromial deltoid; if this line is not visible the muscle is dissected straight from the acromio-clavicular joint for 3-4 cm. If a superior classic approach has been chosen, it is time to make the bony incision on the anterior border of the acromion and to split the future posterior edge of the flap as already described. The flap is elevated and placed on waiting stitches (Fig. 5). Then the cuff is prepared with minimal excision, placing some waiting stitches on the supraspinatus. Behind, the landmark of the posterior edge of the tear is often difficult. A partial bursectomy enhances the visibility. With the help of an Ohman retractor under the acromion the posterior locating stitches are placed. Then the flap is slopped down onto the loss of cuff. Without tying the knots the definite non-absorbable stitches are placed, starting by the posterior corner and the medial edge, then the posterior edge. Those posterior and medial stitches are tied from medial to lateral, releasing the tension with abduction of the arm. The anterior edge can be sutured at the end (Figs. 6 and 7).

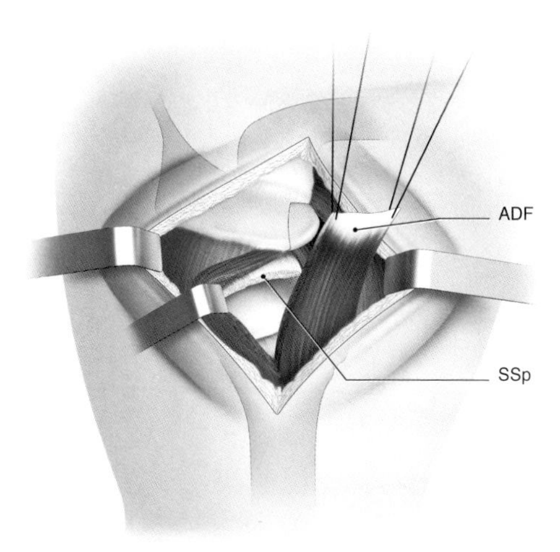

Fig. 5 – The posterior part of the anterior fibres of the deltoid are detached from the acromion.
ADF: Anterior deltoid flap; SSp: Supraspinatus.

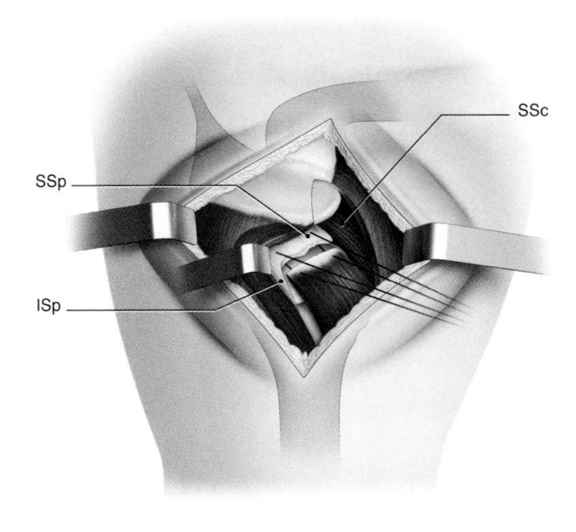

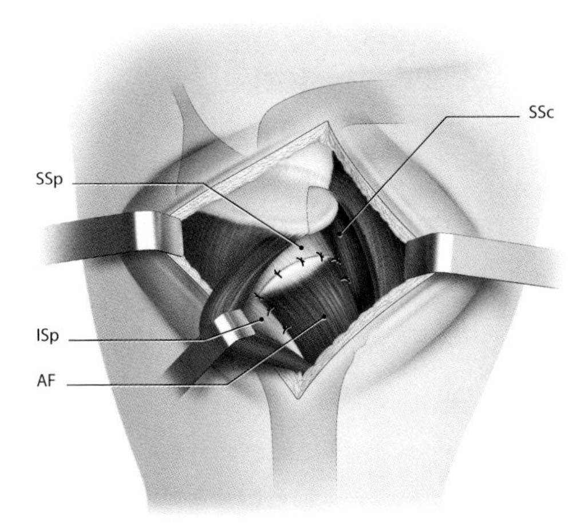

Figs. 6 and 7 – Suture of this flap to the edge of the supraspinatus and infraspinatus. ISp: Infraspinatus; SSp: Supraspinatus; SSc: Subscapularis; AF: Anterior flap.

The closure of the donor site defect is easily done with transosseous knots of the anterior remaining deltoid to the acromion and a continuous suture on the muscular part.

Postoperative management

The patient is placed in an abduction splint at 60° for a 6-week period. The rehabilitation is passively started immediately from the position on the splint and progressive descent after 6 weeks.

Material and methods

Forty-seven patients have been operated on between 1991 and 1994. The mean percentage of the deltoid flap among all rotator cuff tears operations during the same period is 15.4%. None has been lost of view. Thirty-three patients sustained a preliminary study in 1995 (1). Five of them deceased at the time of the second study and one moved away but was contacted and had a good subjective result. Fourteen new cases were added between the two studies. Finally, 41 shoulders were available for this study, with analytic measurements of the active mobility, functional analysis of the Constant-Murley score, and subjective evaluation of the results.

The patients were analyzed into three groups, according to the preoperative deficit of active elevation:

– group 1 < 90°;
– group 2 between 90°and 120°;
– group 3 > 120°.

X-rays evaluation included an AP view in neutral, lateral, and medial rotation, a double oblique view for the measurement of the subacromial space, and a Lamy sagittal radiograph. The degree of arthritis has been quantified according to the Samilson and Priet classification (7). All the patients sustained a preoperative CT scan or an MRI according to the preference of the surgeon. The muscular status has been checked using Goutallier classification for the fatty degeneration (8) and Thomazeau classification for the degree of amyotrophy (9).

The size of the rupture was preoperatively checked as follows:

– in the frontal plane in three stages: lateral, intermediate, or medial retraction;
– in the saggital plane number of tendons involved; one patient sustained an MRI and seven an ultrasonography at the last follow-up.

Results

The final mean follow-up was 7 years (5-8), the average age of the 26 men and 15 women was 59 years (42-78). Thirty-two patients were heavy workers (78%) and 21 still in activity (51%) at the time of surgery. Fourteen had work compensation. Dominant side was involved in 86% of the cases. The average duration of the preoperative period was 10 months. Sixty-five percent had previous rehabilitation and 70% sustained some injections of steroids. Two patients sustained a previous attempt of suturing. The flap was decided preoperatively in 53%. In the coronal plane, the size of the tear was intermediate (stage 2) in 7 cases (17%) and retracted to the glenoid (stage 3) in 34 cases (83%). In the saggital plane, all the patients presented a complete tear of the supraspinatus with a posterior or anterior extension (Table I).

Table I – State of the preoperative lesions in the sagittal plane.

	Sagittal extension					
	Complete SSN	*Complete ISN*	*1/3 sup ISN*	*1/3 sup ISN + SSC*	*Complete ISN + SSC*	*Complete SSC*
n	41 (100%)	21	14	3	1	2

SSN = supraspinatus tendon; ISN = infraspinatus tendon; SSC = suprascapular tendon.

The biceps tendon was involved in 21 cases (52%): 4 subluxated, 6 thick, and 11 disrupted. The rotator interval was involved in 17 cases (41%). On the 16 cases where the fatty degeneration study was available, 12 were stage 3. Acromioplasty was done in all the cases and arthroplasty of the acromio-clavicular joint in 10 cases. Twenty-eight cases were immobilized in abduction at 60°, six with 30°, and seven elbow on body. Post-op rehabilitation was systematic, for 26 (63%) in rehabilitation centers. There was no complication. The average objective final values are shown in Table II.

Table II – Clinical results of the whole series.

	Constant score/100	*Pain/15*	*Active flexion*	*Strength*
Pre-op	37 (12-62)	4.1 (0-12)	113° (0-180)	1.3 (0-6)
Post-op	62 (17-92)	11 (0-15)	148° (30-180)	2.9 (0-11)
p-Value	0.0001	0.0001	0.002	0.002

The mean gain of the Constant score was 25 points and only three patients had lower final score. Four patients had a bad pain result, between 0 and 5 on a 15 points scale. One was already operated on before the flap and the other was the only case of tendon prosthesis of this evaluation. Thirty-eight patients were satisfied or very satisfied (92%) and three not satisfied (8%) because of pain (one case), loss of mobility (one case), or both (one case). Concerning the return to work only 6 (28%) of the 21 still in activity were able to go back to work. The lateral rotation on the 10 points scale of the Constant score increased from 5 to 7 with a high correlation with the active flexion ($p = 0.05$). The distance between the great tuberosity and the acromion was measured in 36 of the 41 cases and decreased from 7.3 mm preoperatively to 5.5 mm at the final review. None was increased, 16 were unchanged (44%) while 20 decreased (56%).

Preoperatively, according to Samilson classification there were 2 cases of arthritis stage 1 and 1 stage 2, while postoperatively 10 were stage 1, 4 stage 2, and 2 stage 3. The presence or absence of radiological arthritis did not influence the final result. One patient, because of a bad painful result, sustained a final MRI and eight patients had an ultrasonography. Among them four flaps were intact with a more than 4 mm thickness and a good final clinical result. In the four cases where the flap appeared thinner than 2 mm (two cases) or disrupted (two cases), the Constant score was lower.

As can be seen in Table III, whatever the group, the patients were not different in age, anatomical lesions, or radiological pre-op status of the cuff lesions. The best gain in Constant score was in group 1 with less pre-op flexion, while the group 3 gained less as much as two of the three failures were from it.

All the patients of group 1 gained in flexion (average 89°, from 10° to 180°). In group 2, one lost 90°, two were unchanged, and nine gained 74.5° (20-100°). On the contrary, in group 3, only four patients increased their final flexion, seven were unchanged (39%), and seven lost 40° in average. This explains the final diminution of flexion of this group (148° against 159° preoperatively).

Table III – Clinical final results according to the degree of preoperative loss of active flexion.

	n	*Age*	*Flexion*	*Pain/15 pts*	*Activities/20*	*Constant score*
			Pre, post	*Pre, post*	*Pre, post*	*Pre, post*
Group 1	11	59.2	46, 144	5.5, 12.2	5.4, 17.2	25, 64
Group 2	12	59.6	103, 151	4.3, 10.6	8.3, 14.6	37, 62
Group 3	18	58	159, 148	3, 10.4	8.5, 15.1	46, 60

Group 1 = flexion less than 90°; group 2 = flexion between 90° and 120°; group 3 = flexion more than 120°.

Chronologic evolution

As previously said, 27 patients have been checked two times using the same methods. This group of 27 patients did not differ from the whole series with an average age of 58 years (42-78) and presented the same lesions. The final follow-up is a little bit higher, 7.4 years (6-8.5). Table IV shows a stable result on pain but an increase in active flexion and strength. On the contrary, the contralateral strength decreased from 7 kg at the first review to 5.8 kg at the last one.

Table IV – Chronological review of the clinical results (n = 27).

	Follow-up (months)	*Constant score*	*Pain*	*Active flexion*	*Strength (kg)*
Preoperative	0	35	4	112°	1
First review	12	58	12	132°	2
Second review	89	64	11.5	150°	3.4

Influence of the age and tear extension

Fourteen patients (34%) were less than 55 years old at the moment of operation. They had the same lesions than the whole series and their follow-up was identical (7 years). Their final Constant score was higher than the whole series (68.9), and the final distance between acromion and great tuberosity was higher, but without statistical significance. The final clinical results were better when the tear involved the posterior cuff than when there was an anterior extension to the subscapularis (only two cases).

Discussion

The deltoid flap in this study gave an average gain of +25 points for the Constant score and 92% of the patients were satisfied. Moreover, strength and active flexion increased with the time. The mean gain in active flexion (+98°) was better for the group with a preoperative pseudoparalytic shoulder. On the contrary, the active flexion decreased in the group with a preoperative flexion of more than 120°.

The deltoid flap is a valuable solution for tears of two tendons or more with preference for posterior extension. A subscapularis tendon involvement is not a good indication for a deltoid flap.

Our results on subjective appreciation and relief of pain were comparable with the other series (10-14). There was some debate in the literature about the efficacy of the deltoid flap in comparison with a simple debridment (10) or about the durability of the results (12). When reading the articles it is also obvious that some differences can be explained by a difference in the extension of the lesions (11). It is important to have a good description of the tear, tendon by tendon in the three plans (15). In this retrospective study, the infraspinatus split was not identified but must be considered as a tear limiting the capability of direct repair. A diminution of the subacromial space and a retraction of the supraspinatus to the glenoid (stage 3) were good indicators of the saggital extension to more than one tendon (14) in as much as the French Society Symposium (16) showed only 5% of isolated tears of the supraspinatus when the tendon was retracted to the glenoid.

The deltoid flaps were decided peroperatively in 53% of our cases when it was not possible to suture the supraspinatus back to the tuberosity with the elbow on body. The difficulty to well define what is an irreparable cuff is also one cause of the divergences found in the published studies. However the progress of the preoperative imaging can help for the decision.

On the contrary to the recent article by Lu et al. (12), our results were better than a simple subacromial decompression which gave, according to the results of the symposium of the French Society of Arthroscopy, for 55-year-old patients, a final Constant score of 65.7 compared to our 68.9 with the deltoid flap (15).

However the decrease of the subacromial space is significant, like others (10, 12), and also the progression of osteoarthritis. This would justify more final imaging than presented here. On the contrary than others (17) there was no case of increase of subacromial space in our series, but a decrease in 56% led to think that our flaps were not anymore functional, even disrupted. This is the classic evolution of any repair as soon as there is more than one tendon involved.

There is actually a consensus around the idea that everything is played according to the pre-op status of the musculo-tendinous unit. The association of retraction, fatty degeneration, muscular atrophy, and tendon split would lead to a rerupture whatever the technique used, but without systematic clinical relevance. It is from the beginning a written story. Our operations allow the patient to overcome the pain period and our technical choices must take account of the advantage for the patient in doing them, especially for difficult techniques with a donor site morbidity or demanding follow-up.

In this point of view the deltoid flap is easy to do with a fair donor site morbidity, can be done with the same incision than a classic repair of a rotator cuff tear. It is however justified to wear an abduction splint for 6 weeks which can be a problem for heavy patients and/or in poor general condition.

Conclusion

The deltoid flap remains a valuable and simple solution for tears of more than one tendon especially for posterior extension to the infraspinatus in young and healthy patients. The pain, strength, and active mobility results are stable even with an important follow-up. It can be decided preoperatively when the imaging shows an alteration of the musculo-tendinous unit such as splitting, fatty degeneration, and muscular atrophy. In fact, whatever the technique used, in these cases of irreparable cuffs, progressive irreversible alteration of the anatomical conditions of the cuff and the glenohumeral joint is often seen over the time, but without systematic clinical relevance.

However it must be avoided when preoperative active flexion is quite normal and when there is no more tendon in front or in the back to suture the edges of the flap.

References

1. Takagishi N (1978) The new operation for the massive rotator cuff rupture. J Jpn Orthop Assoc; 52: 775-780

2. Apoil A, Augereau B (1985) Réparation par lambeau de deltoide des grandes pertes de substance de la coiffe des rotateurs de l'épaule. Chirurgie; 11: 287-290
3. Gerber C, Fuchs B, Hodler J (2000) The results of repair of massive tears of the rotator cuff. J Bone Joint Surg Am; 82: 505-515
4. Thomazeau H, Katz D, Colmar M (1995) Lambeaux deltoidiens, résultats précoces d'une série continue de 35 cas. 8th ESSEC congress, Barcelona. J Shoulder Elbow Surg; 4.1 (part 2) (abstract S28, no. 46)
5. Gedouin JE, Katz D, Colmar M, Thomazeau H, Crovetto N, Langlais F (2002) Deltoid flap for the treatment of massive rotator cuff tear, 41 cases with a mean 7 years follow-up (minimal 5 years). Revue Chir Orthop; 88: 365-372
6. Katz D (2004) Glenoid exposure in total shoulder prosthesis. Revue Chir Orthop; 90: 171-175
7. Samilson RL, Priet V (1983) Dislocation arthropathy of the shoulder. J Bone Joint Surg Am; 65: 456-466
8. Goutallier D, Postel JM, Bernageau J, Voisin MC (1994) Fatty muscle degeneration in cuff ruptures: pre and postoperative evaluation by CT scan. Clin Orthop; 304: 78-83
9. Thomazeau H, Boukobza E, Morcet N, Chaperon J, Langlais F (1997) Prediction of rotator cuff repair results by magnetic resonance imaging. Clin Orthop; 344: 275-283
10. Dierickx C, Vanhoof H (1994) Massive rotator cuff tears treated by a deltoid muscular inlay flap. Acta Orthop Belg; 60: 94-100
11. Le Huec JC, Liquois F, Schaeverbecke T, Zipoli B, Chauvaux, Le Rebeller A (1996) Results of a series of deltoid flaps for the treatment of massive rotator cuff tears with an average follow-up of 3.5 years. Revue Chir Orthop; 82: 22-28
12. Lu XW, Verborgt O, Gazielly D (2008) Long term outcomes after deltoid muscular flap transfer for irreparable rotator cuff tears. J Shoulder Elbow Surg; 17: 732-737
13. Thür C, Jülke M (1995) The anterolateral deltoid muscle flap-plasty: the procedure of choice in large rotator cuff defects. Unfallchiurg; 98: 415-421
14. Vandenbussche E, Bensaida M, mutschler C, Dart T, Augereau B (2004) Massive tears of the rotator cuff treated with a deltoid flap. Int Orthop; 28: 226-230
15. Thomazeau H, Gleyse P, Lafosse L, Walch G, Kelberine F, Coudane H (2000) Arthroscopic assessment of full thickness rotator cuff tears. Arthroscopy; 3: 1-7
16. Kempf JF, Marcillou P, Schlemmer B (1999) Résultats et traitements des ruptures isolées du supraspinatus distales, intermédiaires, et rétractées à la glène. In: Augereau B, Gazielly DF, Les ruptures transfixiantes de la coiffe des rotateurs, Symposium SOFCOT, Revue Chir Orthop; 85: 105-109
17. Spahn G, Kirschbaum S, Klinger HM (2006) A study for evaluating the effect of the deltoid flap repair in massive rotator cuff defects. Knee Surg Sports Traumatol Arthrosc; 14: 365-372

The myotendinous advancements of supra and infraspinatus muscles in the treatment of irreparable retracted tears of the rotator cuff

Ph. Sauzières, J.-M. Postel

Introduction

The large tears of the rotator cuff are considered to be unrepairable when after debridment and surgical release of the ruptured tendons it is not possible to suture them in their anatomic position, or if this suture has to be performed under excessive tension.

This is often the case when the cuff tear involves two or three tendons. The preoperative evaluation of the repairability is based mainly on the analysis of the width of the tendinous gap in the coronal and sagittal planes by the MRI and/or arthro-CT scan. According to the situation of the tendinous stump in the coronal plane (the classifications of Bernageau or Warner), it is considered that a gap of more than 2.5 cm does not allow a direct repair. However, this gap can be related partly to the musculo-tendinous retraction, which can give some elasticity and make the repair easier to perform. It is difficult to evaluate precisely this retraction before surgery, but it is usually found more important in some situations (recent traumatic tear, degenerative tear with low fatty degeneration index (FDI*) inferior to 0.5).

This preoperative evaluation must be made as objectively as possible, in order not to attempt a conventional or arthroscopic direct repair when the risk of re-tear is excessively important.

The anatomical and functional results of the myotendinous advancements depend, as for conventional direct repairs, on the quality of the rotator cuff

---

* The FDI is the sum of the fatty degeneration scores – according to Goutallier and Bernageau's classification – of the three main cuff muscles (supraspinatus, infraspinatus, and subscapularis), divided by 3.

muscles. The FDI must be lower than 2 to have good chances of tendinous healing. If the FDI is ≥2, cuff will re-tear in more than 50% of the cases. Narrowing of the subacromial space (less than 5 mm) is also predictive of poorer anatomical results. It has been found that a negative external rotation elbow alongside (ER1) is associated with a higher risk of re-tear (but ER1 is highly correlated to FDI and narrowing of the subacromial space).

In those desperate situations, it could be better to make the choice of palliative surgery, for instance of a myotendinous transfer (if it is not decided to make a simple debridment). Thus myotendinous advancements are situated between direct tendinous repairs and myotendinous transfers. Although they do not have the notoriety they deserve, they must certainly be included in the therapeutic surgical armentarium of the large rotator cuff tears.

Technique

The myotendinous advancements were described by Jean Debeyre in 1963 for supraspinatus, and by his pupil Daniel Goutallier for infraspinatus in 1972.

Supraspinatus advancement

It is recommended to install the patient in a seated position, but a semi-seated position is usually sufficient (Fig. 1). The operative field includes the entire upper limb, the shoulder, and must incorporate the spinal edge of the scapula and the base of the neck medially. The incision is centered on the lateral edge of the acromion, just anterior to its posterolateral angle (Figs. 2 and 3). It descends on three fingerwidths vertically laterally, and runs medially 1 cm above the spine of the scapula, toward the medial edge of the scapula. The subcutaneous fat is incised to the muscular aponeurosis of the deltoid laterally, and of the trapezius medially (Fig. 4).

Before realising the acromial osteotomy, it is preferable to prepare the holes of the two screws which will be used for the final osteosynthesis of the acromion. Two parallel holes will be drilled at 2.7 mm from the posterior edge of the acromion anteriorly, through the thickness of the acromion, taking care not to penetrate the acromio-clavicular articular space. The acromial osteotomy is made with an oscillating saw, from the lateral edge of the acromion to the junction of the medial edge of the acromion and the spine of the scapula, just behind the acromio-clavicular joint. The opening of the osteotomy can be eased with the use of a Méary retractor, and by releasing the inferior aspect of the acromio-clavicular capsule. The subacromial bursa is then excised to expose the superior aspect of the cuff, particularly of the supraspinatus. Careful hemostasis of the peritendinous fat is needed at this step.

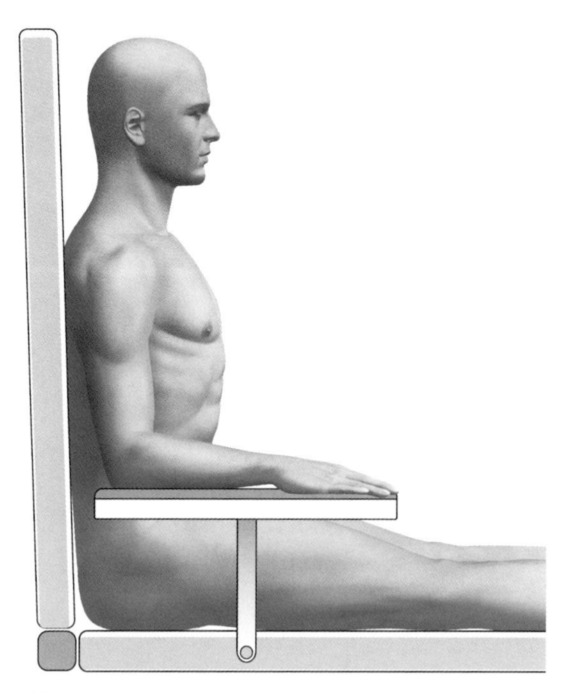

Fig. 1 – Sitting position.

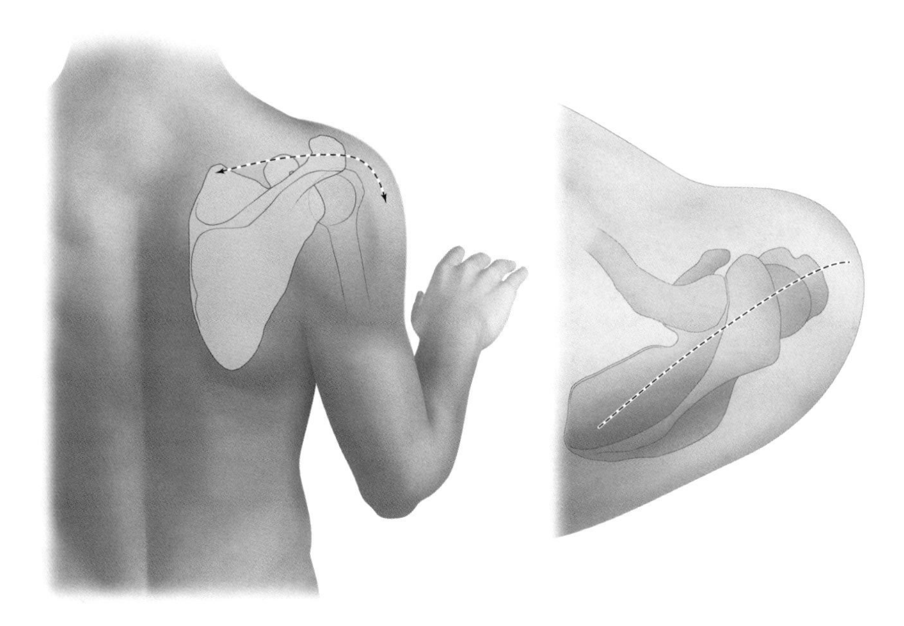

Figs. 2 and 3 – Posteriour-superiour with transacromial approach.

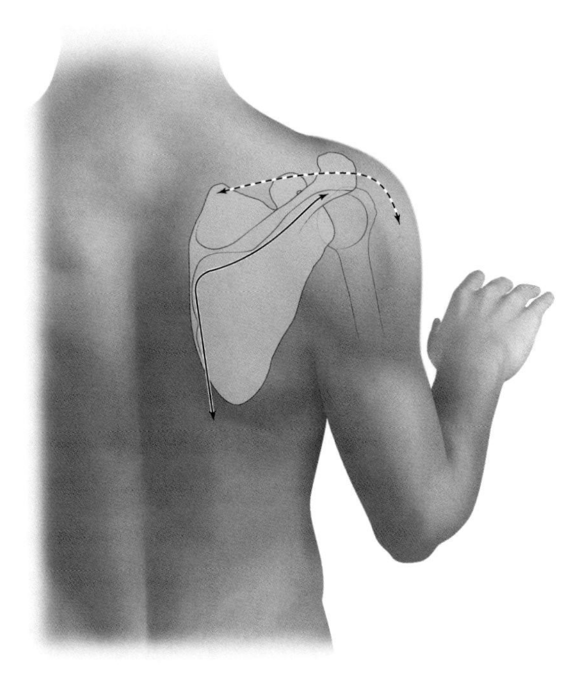

Fig. 4 – Posteriour approach for advancement of infraspinatus.

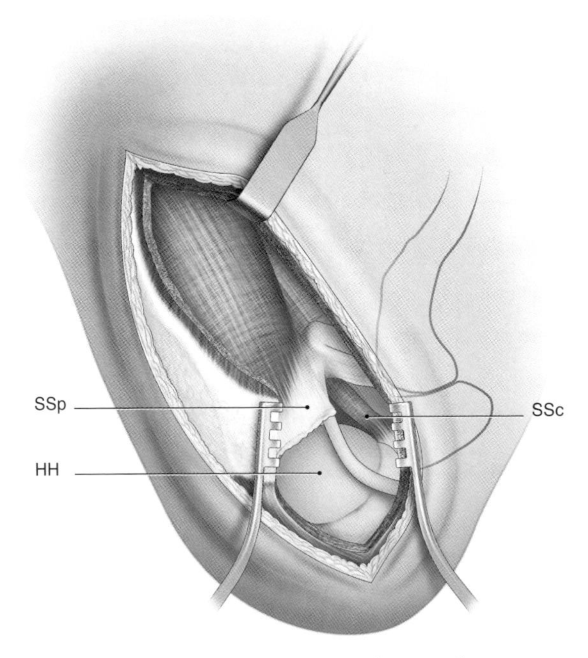

Fig. 5 – Exposition of the lesions through transacromial approach.
SSc: Subscapularis; SSp: Supraspinatus; HH: Humeral head.

The release of the tendinous stump is made from lateral to medial (Fig. 5). Anteriorly, the anterior edge of the tendon must be separated from the rotator interval toward the superior aspect of the coracoid process. Posteriorly the posterior edge of the supraspinatus tendon must be separated from the infraspinatus toward the basis of the spine of the scapula. Medially, the release of the tendon from the upper capsulo-synovial recess must be done carefully because of the vasculo-nervous suprascapular pedicle (Fig. 6). In practice, it is preferable not to go beyond the lateral edge of the foot of the coracoid process.

The release of the muscular body will be performed from medial to lateral with a spatula. The hemostasis of a posterior branch between the pedicle and the lateral edge of the spine of the scapula must be done. The pedicle is raised with the muscle. In order to give more freedom to the pedicle it is highly recommended to cut the white pearly coracoid ligament which closes the notch situated just posterior to the foot of the coracoid process, taking care to preserve the artery situated just anterior and superior to the suprascapular nerve (1).

After the complete release of the musculo-tendinous unit, the lateral mobilization obtained is usually around 2.5-3 cm (Fig. 7). One must check that there is no excessive tension on the pedicle.

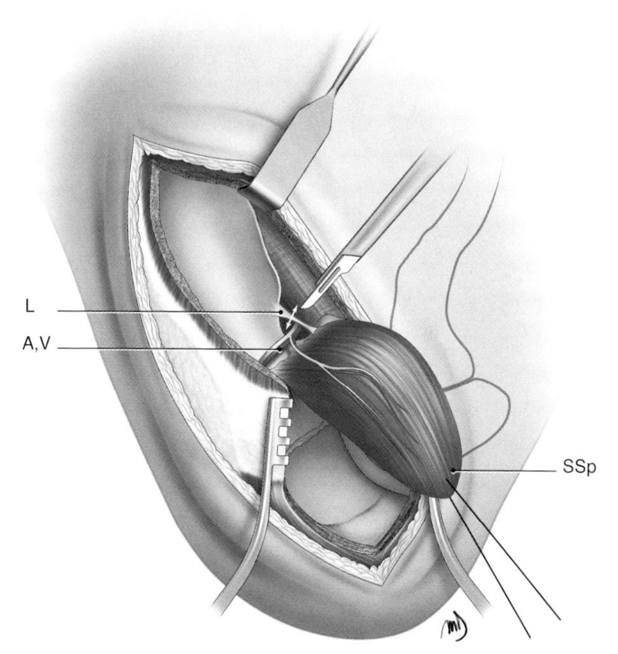

Fig. 6 – Take care of the suprascapular nerve.
A,V: Superior scapular artery, vein; SSp: Supraspinatus; L: *à compléter*

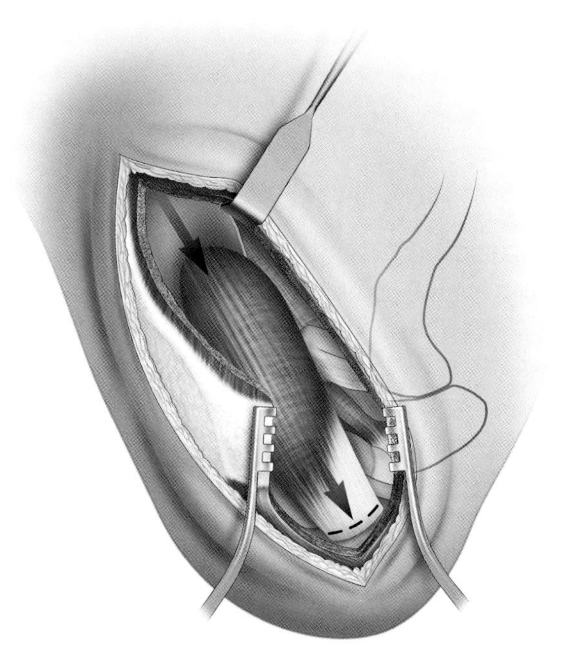

Fig. 7 – Supraspinatus advancement.

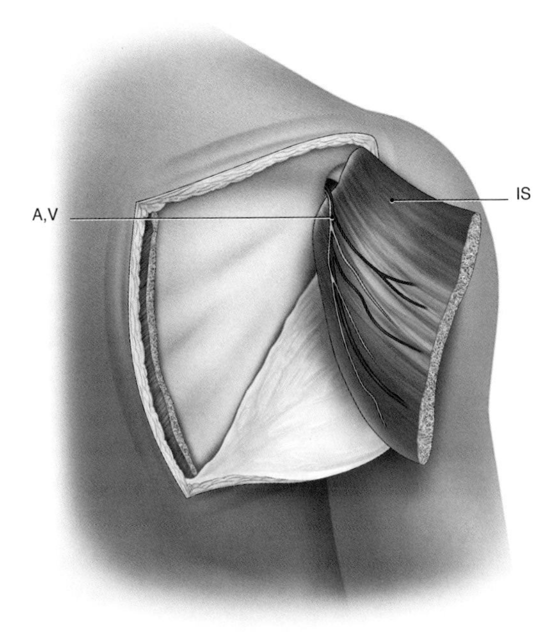

Fig. 8 – Infraspinatus advancement.
ISp: Infraspinatus; SSp: Supraspinatus; SSc: Subscapularis.

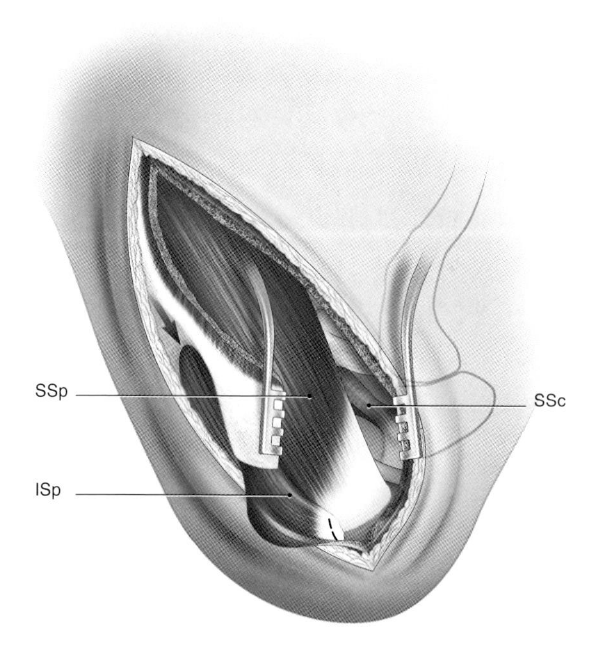

Fig. 9 – Supraspinatus and infraspinatus fix to the footprint.

The tendinous stump will be sutured in a bony trough made at the upper aspect of the greater tuberosity, by two Mason-Allen stitches (Fig. 8). The anterior and posterior edges of the supraspinatus will be sutured to adjacent structures with separated stitches in order to close the cuff.

The muscular body can be fixed to the trapezius in order to put it into some tension.

The closure of the approach necessitates the reduction of the acromiotomy that can be helped by the use of a forceps ("lion's teeth" type, for instance) and its osteosynthesis with two 3.5 mm screws, usually about 40-45 mm long. Titanium screws are usually employed, with washers (Fig. 9).

The upper limb is then positioned on a thoraco-brachial splint in slight abduction for 5 weeks. Passive mobilization is immediately started.

Infraspinatus advancement (Fig. 10)

The infraspinatus advancement needs a completely seated patient, which imposes usually the use of a head support.

The approach is made through a reverse L incision. It begins at the inferior angle of the scapula, goes vertically along the spinal rim of the scapula toward the spine of the scapula, then follows the inferior edge of the spine of the scapula, reaching the posterior head of the deltoid, at about 4 cm below the transacromial approach. An oblique and more direct approach can be done, from inferior to superior and medial to lateral. Then the deeper aspect of the posterior head of the deltoid is released from the infraspinatus muscle, which leads to the infraspinatus tendon. Positioning the arm in abduction makes this step easier. The infraspinatus aponeurosis is incised vertically 2 cm laterally from the spinal rim of the scapula, then along the spine, and finally at the inferior limit of the muscle. The muscle is released from the aponeurotic peripheric flaps until bony contact is reached. The muscular body is ruginated step-by-step from the infraspinatus fossa, laterally and superiorly. At the medial aspect of the inferior edge of the muscle there is a vascular anastomosis between the suprascapular and infrascapular vessels which has to be ligated and cutted. The muscular body is raised to the posterior rim of the glenoid, taking care, when arriving at the spino-glenoid notch, to lift the pedicle and the muscle altogether.

Through the transacromial approach, the infraspinatus is released from the supraspinatus, as previously said, and from the teres minor at its inferior edge. Two Mason-Allen stitches are used to grasp the tendinous stump laterally and help its mobilization. As for supraspinatus, infraspinatus is inserted in a bony trough, without tension. Separated stitches will fix the edges of the infraspinatus to the adjacent tendons.

The muscular body can be sutured to the inferior aponeurotic flap and eventually to the subcutaneous tissues. As an alternative, Goutallier proposes to desinsert the two inferior thirds of the rhomboid major from the spinal edge of the scapula, leaving it in continuity with the infraspinatus aponeurosis, in order to give some tension on the infraspinatus muscle after its release (2).

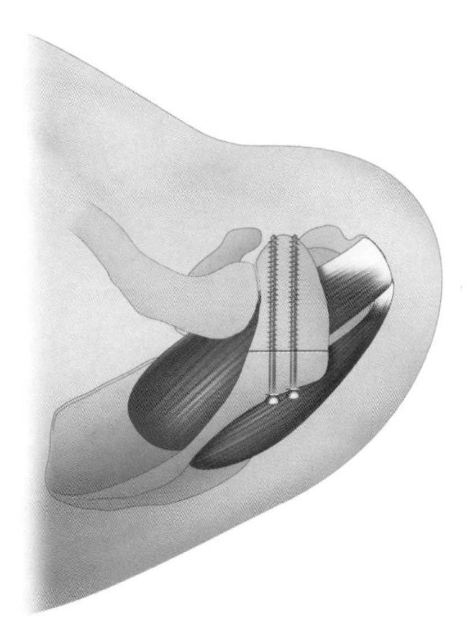

Fig. 10 – Osteosynthesis with two screws of the acromial osteotomy.
IS: Infraspinatus; A,V: Superior scapular artery.

Indications

The myotendinous advancements are used to repair the rotator cuff tears which could not otherwise be closed by direct suture, either conventional or arthroscopic, and where fatty degeneration is not too severe.

Supraspinatus advancements

They can be used in severely retracted tears of the supraspinatus to the glenoid (stage 3), with preservation of a good muscular trophicity (FDI ≤ 1), and without subacromial narrowing.

Infraspinatus advancements

Isolated advancements of the infraspinatus are exceptionally indicated. In theory they are indicated in isolated infraspinatus tears retracted to the glenoid, but usually the importance of the muscular fatty degeneration does not allow such a procedure and a latissimus dorsi transfer will be preferred.

Double supraspinatus and infraspinatus advancements are reserved to the large posterosuperior tears of the rotator cuffs. They suppose a FDI of less than 2, no excessive narrowing of the subacromial space, good anterior active elevation, and no hornblower sign. They can eventually be proposed to young and motivated patients, as postoperative recovery usually takes a long time. They can be opposed to debridements, less ambitious but sometimes wiser, or to latissimus/teres major transfers, as ambitious but more logical when muscles are too heavily degenerated. (The muscle transfers are ambitious but more logical, if you use "as": the advancements are opposed to transfers, as ambitious..., meaning that advancements are ambitious.)

Results (Symposium SO.F.C.O.T 2003) (3)

Review of 30 cases at a mean 5 years follow-up (6 single advancements of the supraspinatus, 24 double advancements)

Constant score raised from 46 preoperatively to 68 at revision, with 8 excellent results (Constant score > 75), 12 good results (Constant score between 65 and 75), and 10 bad results (Constant score <65). Three probable neurodystrophy were noted, one ulnar nerve compression, and no suprascapular nerve problem. Two arthroscopic tenotomies of the long head of the biceps had to be performed secondarily.

Arthro-CT scan controls found 79% of watertight cuffs at follow-up, and 21% re-tears.

Constant score was better for the intact cuffs (71) than for the cuffs with re-tears (63).

The predictive factors of re-tear were:

- High FDI:
  - FDI < 2: 91% watertight cuffs
  - FDI ≥ 2: 43% re-tears
- Subacromial distance narrowing (SAD):
  - SAD ≥ 5 mm: 91% watertight cuffs
  - SAD < 5 mm: 66% re-tears
- Impaired active external rotation elbow alongside (ER1):
  - ER1 < 20°: 40% re-tears

References

1. Goutallier D, Postel JM, Boudon R, Lavaul L, Bernageau J (1996) Etude du risque neurologique à l'avancement tendinomusculaire des supra-épineux et infra-épineux dans les réparations des larges ruptures de coiffe. Rev Chir Orthop; 82: 299-305
2. Goutallier D, Postel JM, Van Driessche S, Godefroy D, Radier C (2006) Tension-free cuff repairs with excision of macroscopic tendon lesions and muscular advancement: results in a prospective series with limited fatty muscular degeneration. J Shoulder Elbow Surg; 15: 164-172
3. Postel JM, Goutallier D, Baldoncini J (2004) Traitement des ruptures associées des supra-épineux et infra-épineux par sutures après avancement tendino-musculaire. Rev Chir Orthop; 90 (suppl. 5): 154-170

Pectoralis major transfer: surgical anatomy, technique of harvesting, methods of fixation, postoperative management

A. Kilinc, Ph. Valenti

Surgical anatomy

The pectoralis major muscle (PM) is a broad, thick, triangular muscle situated at the upper and fore part of the chest, anterior to the axilla.

Origin

The origin of the PM is composed by two heads: clavicular and sternocostal. The clavicular head arises from the medial half of the clavicle, while the sternocostal head from the anterior and lateral manubrium, the body of the sternum, the aponeurosis of external oblique muscle, and upper seven costal cartilages (not always the first and the seventh) (Fig. 1).

Direction

From this extensive origin the fibers converge toward their insertion; those arising from the clavicle pass obliquely downward and lateralward, and are usually separated from the rest by a slight interval; those from the lower part of the sternum, and the cartilages of the lower true ribs, run upward and lateralward; while the middle fibers pass horizontally.

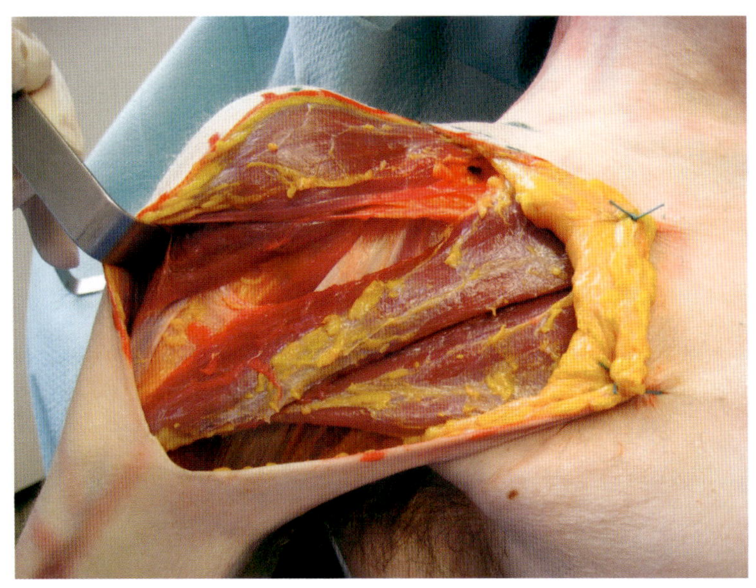

Fig. 1 – PM clavicular and sternocoastal heads.

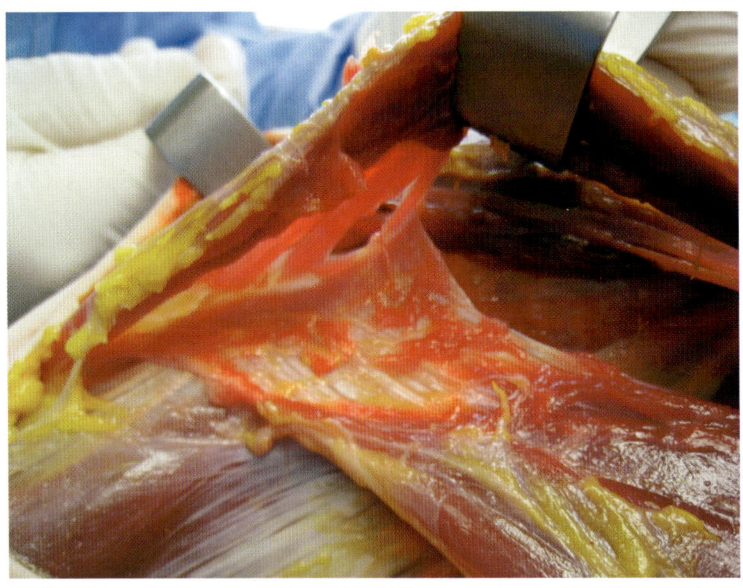

Fig. 2 – The PM tendon appears to be twisted. The posterior lamina of the tendon receives the attachment of the sternal portion. This lamina ascends higher, turning backward successively behind the superficial.

Insertion

All the fibers end on the lateral part of the bicipital groove by a broad tendon (about 5 cm). This tendon consists of two laminæ, placed one in front of the other, and usually blended together below. The anterior lamina (thicker) receives the clavicular fibers. The posterior lamina of the tendon receives the attachment of the sternal portion. These deep fibers, and particularly those from the lower costal cartilages, ascend the higher, turning backward successively behind the superficial and upper ones, so that the tendon appears to be twisted (horseshoe-shaped cross-section). During elevation, the tendon becomes untwisted (Fig. 2).

Innervation

The PM is innervated by the lateral and medial pectoral nerves respectively for the clavicular and the sternal heads (C5-C6 for the clavicular head and C7-C8-T1 for the sternocostal head). These nerves course from a superior to inferior direction and enter the muscle along its posterior surface. The innervation can be jeopardized during dissection if the medial release is too extensive (Fig. 3).

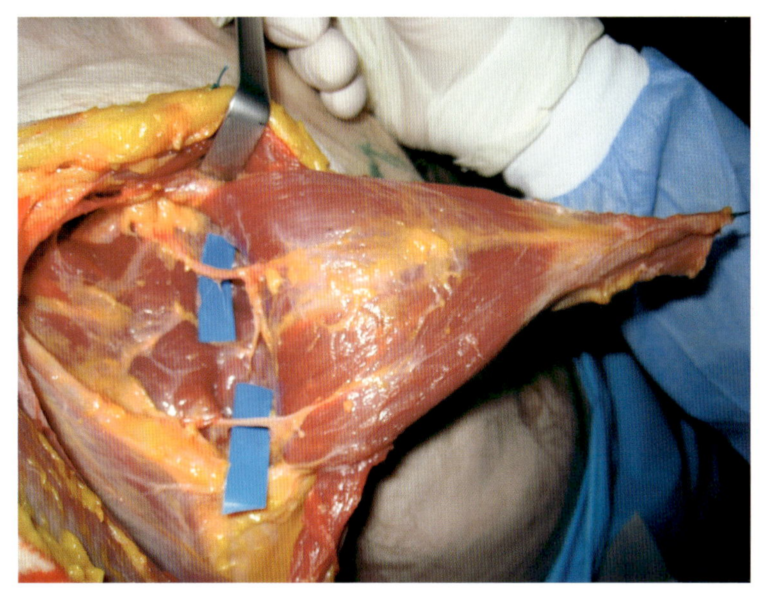

Fig. 3 – Lateral and medial pectoral nerves. The medial release should not exceed 10 cm from the tendon.

Vascularization

The arterial supply is given by the pectoral branch of the thoraco-acromial trunk. The vascularization of the clavicular part of the PM is independent from the sternocostal part (1).

Action

The pectoralis major has three actions. It flexes, adducts, and medially rotates the humerus.

Technique of harvesting and methods of fixation

Installation

Surgery is performed under general anesthesia with an interscalene block to manage postoperative pain. The patient is placed in beach chair position on the border of the surgical table to allow a complete access to the shoulder (2-4). An articulated hydraulic arm holder can be used but usually the arm is simply placed in an arm-rest without any traction. The bony landmarks of the shoulder are palpated and outlined.

Approach

An extended delto-pectoral approach is performed (12-14 cm) from the tip of the coracoid process to inferior border of the bicipital groove. The interval between the anterior deltoid and the PM is developed. The cephalic vein is retracted laterally with the deltoid muscle while the conjoined tendon is retracted medially.

Dissection and cuff assessment

With the arm in abduction and internal rotation, all the adhesions and the scar tissues due to previous surgeries are released in the subacromial space and around the lesser tuberosity.

The superior and anterior rotator cuff is assessed and the tendon of the biceps is identified. According to its aspect and the age of the patient, the long head of the biceps can be tenotomized or tenodesed in the bicipital groove (with a suture anchor or an interference screw).

The anterior humeral circumflex vessels are cauterized. The axillary nerve is identified and protected during the surgery but it is not necessary to place any loop around the nerve.

An attempt is always made to repair the subscapularis tendon. The tendon is identified and grasped with a non-absorbable suture with using a modified Mason-Allen technique. The subscapularis is released from the rotator interval, the coraco-humeral ligament and the neck of the scapula. If the subscapularis tendon is partially or not reparable, a PM transfer is then performed. Often the inferior third of the subscapularis tendon is reparable and the PM transfer is used to improve the repair and the postoperative strength (5).

PM tendon transfer

The inferior and superior borders of the PM are identified at the level of the humerus. According to the size of the repair, the quality of tendon, or the surgeon preferences, the PM can be totally or partially transferred (sternocostal head transfer or clavicular head transfer) (2, 4).

- *Entire tendon transfer:* The PM is entirely harvested, released, and tagged with non-absorbable braided sutures. The tendon is passed over the conjoined tendon toward the lesser tuberosity (2).
- *Sternocostal head transfer:* Only the sternalcostal head is harvested and transferred (6). The interval between the sternal and the clavicular heads of the PM is developed. The sternal head is harvested from the humerus and the muscle is splitted medially (never more than 10 cm to avoid nerve damage). The tendon is tagged with non-absorbable sutures and passed over or underneath the clavicular head and repaired to the lesser tuberosity (4) (Fig. 4).
- *Clavicular head transfer:* Sometimes it is difficult to separate both parts of the tendon, but the clavicular tendinous fibers are superficial and inferior located. Once the tendon is identified, the tendon is tagged with sutures and passed over the tip of the coracoid toward the lesser tuberosity (7). The proximal two-thirds of the tendon can also be taken. In this situation, the fibers from the abdominal portion (from external oblique muscle) have to be transected (3).

Recent studies have shown that passing the tendon underneath (Fig. 5) the conjoint tendon is interesting in terms of strength due to a pulley effect but must be performed gently after dissection of the musculo-cutaneous nerve (8-10). The PM tendon should pass inferiorly and posterior to the musculo-cutaneous nerve. A coracoidoplasty can be necessary to avoid impingement between the PM tendon and the tip of the coracoid process.

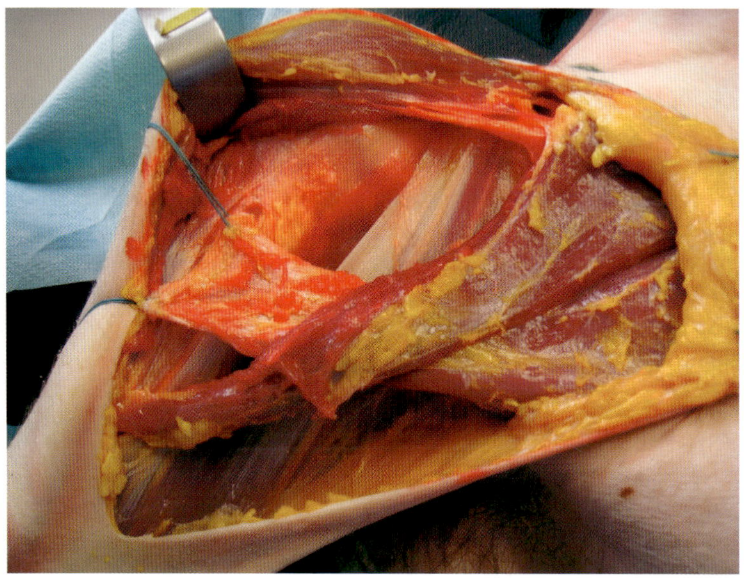

Fig. 4 – The sternocostal head is harvested and tag sutured before passing under the clavicular head.

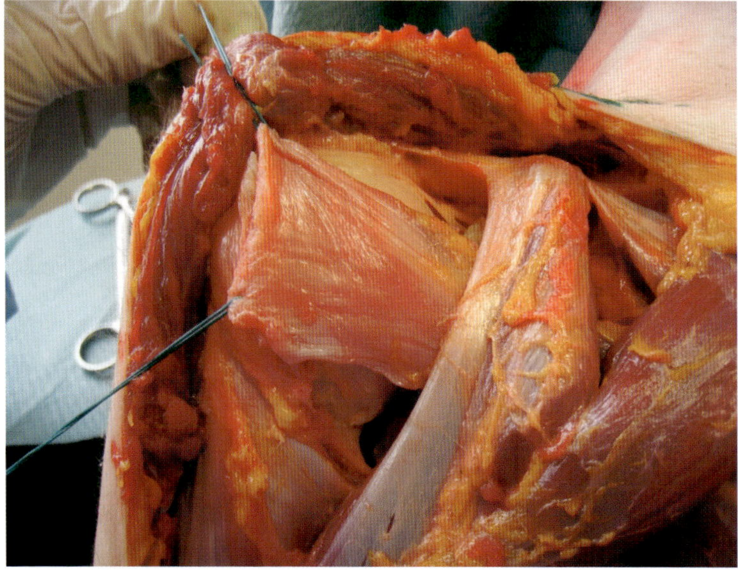

Fig. 5 – The PM transfer is made underneath the conjoint tendon after gentle dissection. A coracoidoplasty may be necessary.

Tendon fixation

The area of fixation on the lesser tuberosity is decorticated and the tendon of the PM is fixed transosseously to the bone (with two 2.7 mm tunnels) or with suture anchors. The use of non-absorbable braided suture is recommended. Some authors (2, 4) recommend reinforcement of the fixation with a thin titanium plate (Stratec/Synthes, Paoli, PA) or repairing the tendon transosseously into a bony trough that is prepared with a high speed burr.

The supraspinatus tendon is sutured to the proximal border of the pectoralis major tendon, to close the rotator interval. The tendon is sutured with the arm between 0° and 30° of external rotation. A drainage is always used. Fixation is tested before skin closure (Fig. 5).

Postoperative management

The patient is immobilized in a sling with the arm at the side in neutral position during 6 weeks. Postoperative pain is managed with an interscalene pump. Passive range of motion is started early with a physiotherapist. Aquatherapy is started after stitches removal. Passive external rotation over 30° is allowed after 4 weeks and an active rehabilitation after 6 weeks. Strengthening exercises are delayed for 6 months.

References

1. Chaffai MA, Mansat M (1988) Anatomic basis for the construction of a musculotendinous flap derived from the pectoralis major muscle. Surg Radiol Anat; 10(4): 273-282
2. Jost B, Puskas GJ, Lustenberger A, Gerber C (2003) Outcome of pectoralis major transfer for the treatment of irreparable subscapularis tears. J Bone Joint Surg Am; 85A(10): 1944-1951
3. Resch H, Povacz P, Ritter E, Matschi W (2000) Transfer of the pectoralis major muscle for the treatment of irreparable rupture of the subscapularis tendon. J Bone Joint Surg Am; 82(3): 372-382
4. Warner JJ (2001) Management of massive irreparable rotator cuff tears: the role of tendon transfer. Instr Course Lect; 50: 63-71
5. Elhassan B, Ozbaydar M, Massimini D, Diller D, Higgins L, Warner JJP (2008) Transfer of pectoralis major for the treatment of irreparable tears of subscapularis: does it work? J Bone Joint Surg Br; 90(8): 1059-1065

6. Jennings GJ, Keereweer S, Buijze GA, De Beer J, DuToit D (2007) Transfer of segmentally split pectoralis major for the treatment of irreparable rupture of the subscapularis tendon. J Shoulder Elbow Surg; 16(6): 837-842
7. Vidil A, Augereau B (2000) Transfer of the clavicular portion of the pectoralis major muscle in the treatment of irreparable tears of the subscapularis muscle. Rev Chir Orthop Reparatrice Appar Mot; 86(8): 835-843
8. Klepps SJ, Goldfarb C, Flatow E, Galatz LM, Yamaguchi K (2001) Anatomic evaluation of the subcoracoid pectoralis major transfer in human cadavers. J Shoulder Elbow Surg; 10(5): 453-459
9. Konrad GG, Kreuz P, Suedkamp N, Jolly J, McMahon P, Debski R (2007) Pectoralis major tendon transfers above or underneath the conjoint tendon in subscapularis-deficient shoulders. An in vitro biomechanical analysis. J Bone Joint Surg Am; 89(11): 2477-2484
10. Galatz LM, Connor PM, Calfee RP, Hsu JC, Yamaguchi K (2003) Pectoralis major transfer for anterior-superior subluxation in massive rotator cuff insufficiency. J Shoulder Elbow Surg; 12(1): 1-5

Transfer of the pectoralis major for the treatment of irreparable subscapularis tear: review of 15 cases

Ph. Valenti, J. Kany, S. Ferriere, A. Kilinc, L. Thomsen

Introduction

Rupture of the subscapularis tendon is rare compared with the tears of supraspinatus and infraspinatus tendons. Involvement of subscapularis tendon has been reported in only 3.5-8% of rotator cuff tear (1-3). Lesion of the subscapularis are isolated (2, 4) or associated with a massive cuff tear (5-7) or occurred after a recurrent anterior dislocation of the shoulder (8-10). In young patient, a trauma in extreme external rotation with the arm in adduction can be found (11). The symptoms are not specific, frequently well tolerated with only a weakness shoulder and an inconstant pain on the anterior area of the shoulder. These factors can explain a delay to make the diagnosis. An acute lesion misdiagnosed becomes a chronic rupture with an atrophic muscle and fatty degeneration of the subscapularis muscle (>stage 3 according to the Goutallier classification (12)). A chronic tear, with a tendon retracted at the level of the glenoid cannot be repaired anatomically or with tension and a high risk of recurrent tear. Thus, tendon transfer can be an option and many techniques have been described: Gerber and Krushell (11) used the third superior part of the PM and transferred it over the coracoids; Jost et al. (13) detached the entire tendon of the PM and brought it over the coracoids; Resch et al. (14) used the clavicular head of the PM which is rerouted underneath the conjoined tendon to try to reproduce the line of action of the subscapularis. The aim of this current study was to report clinical results of clavicular head (eight cases) or sternal head (seven cases) rerouted underneath the conjoined tendon in irreparable subscapularis tear.

Material and methods

Between 2002 and 2007, 15 consecutive pectoralis major tendon transfers were performed by two surgeons (Ph.V. and J.K.) for irreparable subscapularis tendon tear. All patients had given written, informed consent before undergoing this procedure. In all cases, direct tendon repair without tension was impossible regarding the degree of retraction of the tendon or the bad quality of the tendon or the poor elasticity of the muscle after release. All the patients did not respond with conservative treatment combined physiotherapy and injection of corticosteroid drug for a duration of at least 3-6 months. Ten men and five women were operated with an average age of 57 years old (range 37-66 years old). The dominant arm was involved in eight cases (60%). Nine patients were manual workers and six patients were retired with a sedentary daily activity. Nine patients sustained a traumatic event in which three patients with a history of traumatic anterior dislocation followed by recurrent anterior instability. Three shoulders had an isolated subscapularis tear and 12 had a concomitant tear of the supraspinatus tendon. Seven patients had previous surgery: one had had a bone block anteriorly and posteriorly for post-traumatic instability and complained a weakness shoulder; six were failed a massive cuff repair and two of the six failed a subscapularis repair. The average interval from the traumatic event to the pectoralis major transfer was 21 months (range 5-6 months). All the patients complained an anterior shoulder pain with a loss of strength particularly in medial rotation. Sometimes the pain radiated into the medial part of the arm and evocated a pathology of the long head of the biceps.

Functional assessment of the shoulder used the elements of Constant and Murley score (15). Diagnosis of rupture of the subscapularis can be strongly evocated with a clinical examination. Passive external rotation the arm at the side was greater than in the controlateral health side. The lift off test described by Gerber and Krushell (11) was always positive (patients were unable to maintain the raised position of the hand behind the back). Belly press test (16) was positive in all patients (patient was unable to maintain the elbow anteriorly when he exerted a pressure on the stomach). To measure the force in abduction in 90° with extension of the elbow in kilograms, we used a spring balance. In this retrospective series we did not measure postoperatively the strength the upper limb adducted with the elbow in 90° of flexion or during the lift off test (14).

Standard radiographs and computed tomography (CT scan) or magnetic resonance imaging (MRI) with arthrography allowed us a preoperative radiological assessment. Anteroposterior and outlet view assessed a static or a dynamic anterosuperior migration with an escape of the humeral head underneath the coraco-acromial arch, which is a formal contraindication of pectoralis major transfer. An axillary view can detect a static anterior instability (17). Atrophy muscle and fatty infiltration of the rotator cuff was analyzed with Computed tomography (10 cases) or MRI (5 cases) with arthrography regarding Goutallier classification (12). An ultrasonography was performed for five patients with the goal to define the size of the avulsion of the subscapularis tendon in sagittal plane (18), a concomitant lesion of the long head of the biceps and the status of the suprapinatus.

Preoperatively the subscapularis tendon was completely detached from the less tuberosity in 15 cases but in 3 cases the inferior portion of tendon was still attached. Rupture of the supraspinatus tendon was associated in 12 cases and retracted at the level of the glenoid in 6 cases. The mean global fatty degeneration index (GFDI) was 3.24 for the subscapularis and 1.75 for the supraspinatus muscle (12). Six cases had preoperatively a documented information of the long head of the biceps: three were dislocated, two were intact, and one was inflammatory.

Indications and contraindications

Pectoralis major transfer is indicated preoperatively for rupture of the subscapularis tendon retracted at the level of the glenoid and with a muscle infiltrated grade III or IV (12, 19). Indication should be confirmed intraoperatively. Sometimes it is possible to perform a partial repair of the subscapularis remaining component (lower portion) and this repair increases the efficiency of the tendon transfer.

Pseudoparalytic shoulder secondary to a deficiency of the coraco-acromial arch and with a static or a dynamic superior and anterior migration of the humeral head is a contraindication of PM transfer. Chronic anterior dislocation or glenohumeral joint (20), with a pseudoparalytic shoulder, is a candidate for a reverse shoulder prosthesis.

Anatomical surgery

Anatomical dissection in fresh cadavers should be recommended before to perform a pectoralis major transfer. Dissection should focus to the position of the musculo-cutaneous and axillary nerve, and the location of the neurovascular pedicle that supply the PM. The musculo-cutaneous nerve runs medially to the coracoid process under the pectoralis minor before to penetrate into the conjoint tendon muscle. The distance between the coracoid process and the main trunk of the musculo-cutaneous nerve as it entered the coracobrachialis averaged 6.1 cm (3.5-10 cm). The distance between the proximal branch of the musculo-cutaneous nerve for the coraco-brachialis tendon and the coracoid process averaged 4.4 cm (2.1-9 cm) (21).

The axillary nerve from the posterior trunk runs over the anterior muscular portion of the subscapularis before lies superior to the aponeurosis of the latissimus dorsi. Axillary nerve should be identified before to release the remaining of the inferior part of the subscapularis. Circumflex artery and vein should be ligated during the dissection of the axillary nerve.

The PM is innervated by the lateral and medial pectoral nerves respectively for the clavicular and the sternal heads (C5-C6 for the clavicular head and C7-C8-T1 for the sternocostal head). These nerves course from a superior to inferior direction and enter the muscle along its posterior surface. The lateral pectoral nerve penetrates into the deep part of the clavicular head 12.5 cm from the humeral insertion. The medial pectoral nerve penetrates into the deep part of the sternal head 8.5 cm from the humeral insertion and 2 cm from the inferior border. The innervation can be jeopardized during dissection if the medial release is too extensive. A safe distance of 8.5 cm from the insertion of PM to the humerus should be respected to avoid any damage of the innervation of the tendon transfer. Musculo-cutaneous nerve should not only be palpated but also be visualized on transfer to verify that adequate space is present for passage superficial to the nerve.

Surgical technique

Surgery was performed in beach chair position under general anesthesia with an interscalenic block. A subclavicular catheter was left during 24 hours to manage postoperative pain. An extended delto-pectoral approach (12-15 cm) allowed to assess anterosuperior cuff and to harvest pectoralis major tendon (Fig. 1). The cephalic vein was retracted laterally with the anterior fibers of the deltoid and the conjoined tendon was retracted medially. With the arm in abduction and medial rotation, the scar tissue over the less tuberosity was resected, and the stump of the subscapularis retracted under the conjoined tendon was identified and grasped with two non-absorbable sutures (Fig. 2). In seven cases, the shoulder had been previously operated, and we dissected and identified systematically the musculo-cutaneous and axillary nerve to prevent any nerve damage (Fig. 3). During the release of adhesions and the resection of bursa, capsule, and scar tissue over the less tuberosity, we ligated the anterior humeral circumflex artery. The remaining subscapularis tendon was released from the rotator interval, the coraco-humeral ligament, and the neck of the scapula, and an attempt was always made to repair it. In three cases the inferior third of the subscapularis tendon was preserved and the PM transfer was used to improve the repair and the postoperative strength (22). When the long head of the biceps was assessed preoperatively subluxated or dislocated medially or inflammatory, regarding the age and the aspect of the tendon, we performed a tenotomy or a tenodesis (with a suture anchor or an interference screw). In 12 cases, the supraspinatus tendon was torn and reparable after release in 6 cases. When the supraspinatus tendon was irreparable (six cases) the PM tendon transfer was fixed to the anterior part of the great tuberosity.

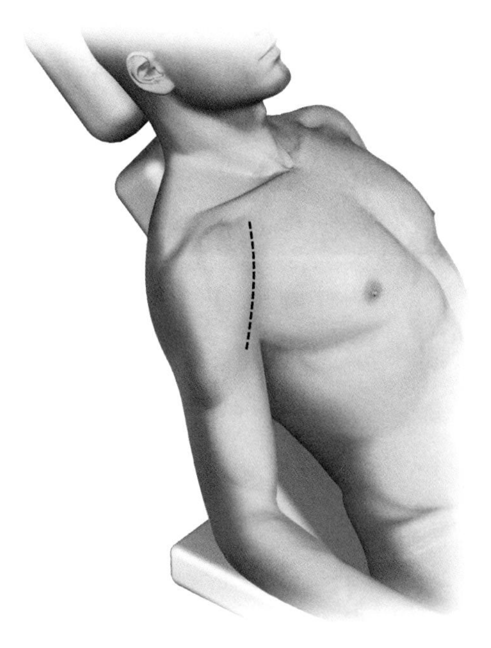

Fig. 1 – Delto pectoral aproach extended distally to the arm.

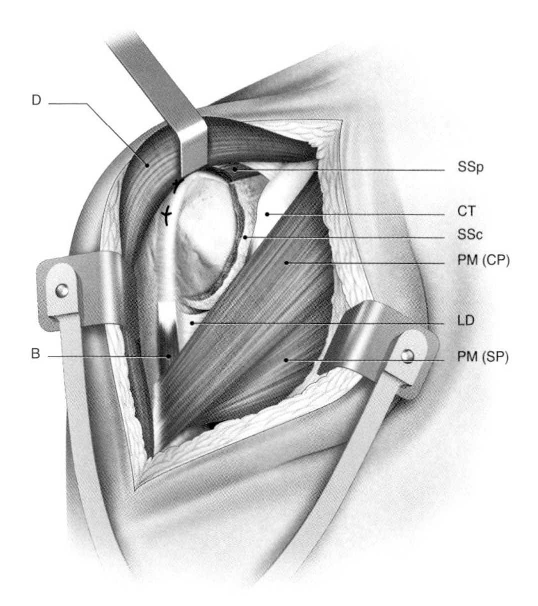

Fig. 2 – Subscapularis retracted atrophic and unreductible.
D: Deltoid muscle; SSp: Supraspinatus; CT: Conjoint tendon; SSc: Subscapularis; B: Biceps; PM (CP): Pectoralis major (clavicular part); PM (SP): Pectoralis major (sternal part); LD: Latissimus dorsi.

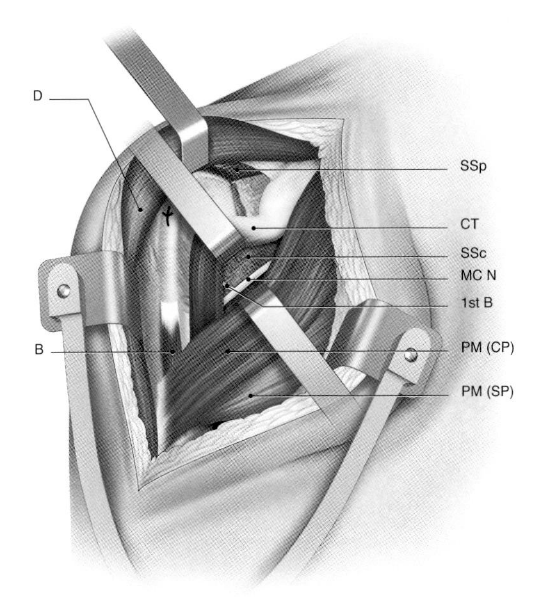

Fig. 3 – Musculo cutaneous nerve should be dissected inside the coracoid process.
D: Deltoid muscle; SSp: Supraspinatus; CT: Conjoint tendon; SSc: Subscapularis; MC N: Musculocutaneous nerve; 1st B: 1st branch; B: Biceps; PM (CP): Pectoralis major (clavicular part); PM (SP): Pectoralis major (sternal part); LD: Latissimus dorsi.

The tendon of the pectoralis major was exposed at the level of the humerus in front of the long head of the biceps. Two types of tendon transfers were harvested in our series (Figs. 4 and 5): eight clavicular head and seven sternal head of the PM. An interval can be found easily and facilitate the dissection of these two heads. The sternal head that was inserted underneath the clavicular head was detached with periosteum and cortical bone from the humerus. A gentle medially dissection of the sternal part should be limited at 10 cm from the humerus and 2 cm from the inferior border of the tendon to avoid nerve damage. The sternal tendon was tagged with non-absorbable suture and passed underneath the clavicular head. A way was created under the conjoined tendon with the musculo-cutaneous nerve posteriorly.

The clavicular tendinous fibers are superficial and inferior located. Once the tendon is identified, the tendon is tagged with sutures and passed under the coracoids process.

Recent studies have shown that passing the tendon transfer underneath the conjoint tendon is interesting in terms of strength due to a pulley effect but must be performed gently after dissection of the musculo-cutaneous nerve (21). The PM tendon should pass anteriorly to the musculo-cutaneous nerve. A coracoidoplasty can be necessary if the tendon transfer is too bulky, to avoid impingement between the PM tendon and the tip of the coracoid process.

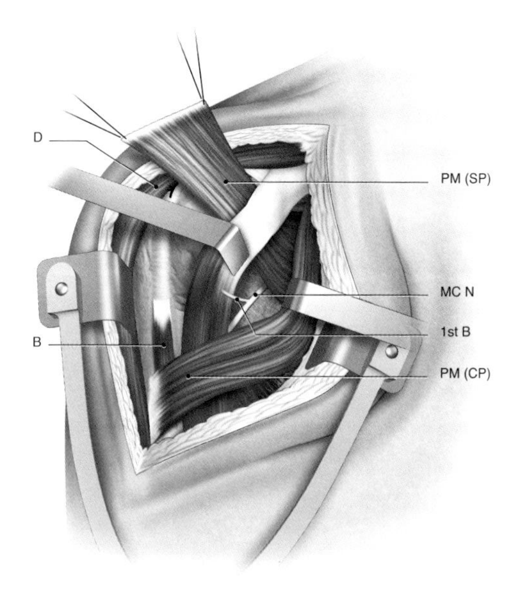

Fig. 4 – Sternal head of the pectoralis major with an oblique direction is passed under the conjoint tendon.
Be careful to the musculo cutaneous nerve.
D: Deltoid muscle; B: Biceps; PM (SP): Pectoralis major (sternal part); MC N: Musculocutaneous nerve; 1st B: 1st branch; PM (CP): Pectoralis major (clavicular part).

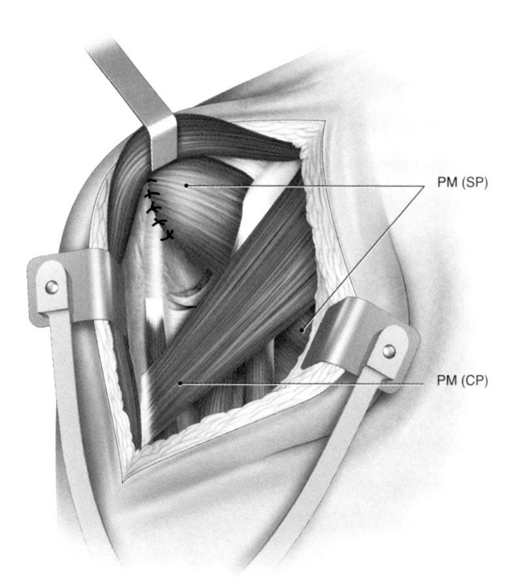

Fig. 5 – Fixation of the sternal head to the anterior part of the foot print and the less tuberosity sharpened.
PM (CP): Pectoralis major (clavicular part); PM (SP): Pectoralis major (sternal part).

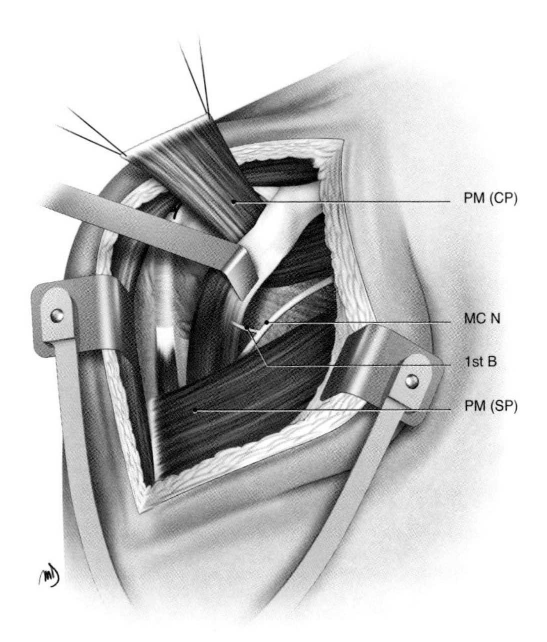

Fig. 6 – Clavicular head with an horizontal direction under the conjoined tendon.
PM (CP): Pectoralis major (clavicular part); PM (SP): Pectoralis major (sternal part); MC N: Musculocutaneous nerve; 1st B: 1st branch.

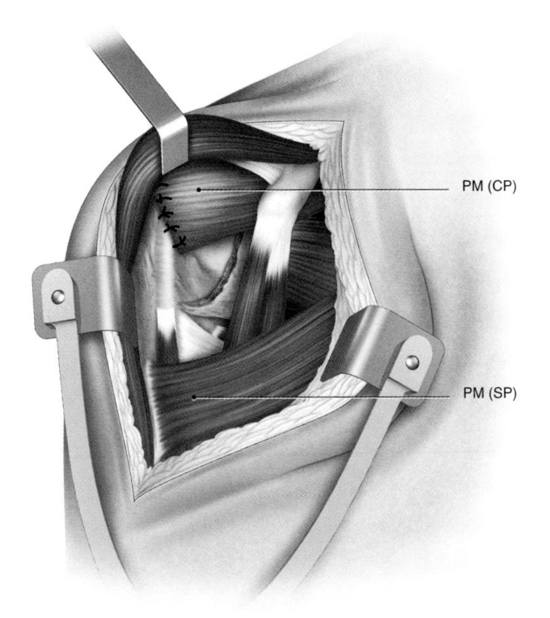

Fig. 7 – Fixation to the less tuberosity of the clavicular head.
PM (CP): Pectoralis major (clavicular part); PM (SP): Pectoralis major (sternal part).

Tendon fixation (Figs. 6 and 7)

The area of fixation onto the lesser tuberosity was decorticated and the tendon of the PM was fixed transosseously to the bone (with two 2.7 mm tunnels) or with suture anchors. The use of non-absorbable braided suture is recommended. Some authors (13, 23) recommend reinforcement of the fixation with a thin titanium plate (Stratec/Synthes, Paoli, PA) or repairing the tendon transosseously into a bony trough that is prepared with a high speed burr. The supraspinatus tendon is sutured to the proximal border of the pectoralis major tendon, to close the rotator interval.

The tendon is sutured with the arm between 0° and 30° of external rotation. A drainage is always used. Fixation is tested before skin closure.

Postoperative management

The patient is immobilized in a sling with the arm at the side in neutral position during 6 weeks. Postoperative pain is managed with an interscalene pump. Passive range of motion is started early with a physiotherapist. Aquatherapy is started after stitches removal. Passive external rotation over 30° is allowed after 4 weeks and an active rehabilitation after 6 weeks. Strengthening exercises are delayed for 6 months.

Results

At an average follow-up of 24 months (range 12-50 months), nine patients were very satisfied, three were satisfied, and three were dissatisfied. In the global series (Table I), the mean absolute Constant score increased from 36 preoperatively to 60 height at the latest follow-up. The score for pain improved with an average of 3 points preoperatively to 14 postoperatively (gain of 11 points; $p < 0.001$). The gain of active forward elevation and external rotation were limited: active forward elevation increased from an average of 140° preoperatively (range 60-170°) to 150° postoperatively (range 60-180°). Active external rotation the arm at the side (ER1) increased an average of 36° preoperatively (range 20-60°) to 42° postoperatively (range 30-80°). The mean postoperative Constant score of medial rotation was 7: eight patients were able to reach the lumbar spine with the thumb and four could touch the sacrum. Strength testing was performed at 90° of abduction in the plane of the scapula. We excluded one patient with an active forward elevation less than 60°. The abduction strength improved from an average of 0.750 kg (range 0-4 kg) preoperatively to an average of 2.250 kg (range 1-5 kg) at the latest follow-up.

Table I – Results of pre- and postoperative clinical examination of the 15 patients*

	Preoperative	*Postoperative*	*Gain*
Pain (15 points)	3 (0-10)	14 (10-15)	11
Daily activities (*20 points*)	7 (0-14)	13 (6-17)	6
Active flexion (*degrees*)	*140* (60-170)	150 (60-180)	10
Active external rotation (*degrees*)	36 (20-60)	42 (30-80)	6
Active internal rotation (10 points)	3 (0-8)	7 (4-8)	4
Strength (*20 points*)	3 (0-16)	9 (4-20)	6
At 90° of flexion absolute Constant score (*100 points*)	36 (22-76)	68 (41-88)	32

*The values are given as the average and the range.

Table II – Pre- and postoperative clinical results. The two groups of PM transfer: group 1: sternal head of PM, group 2: clavicular head of PM*

	Preoperative	*Postoperative*	*Gain*
Group 1: sternal head of PM, *n* = 7 cases			
Pain (*15 points*)	6	14	8
Daily activities (*20 points*)	8	14	6
Active flexion (*degrees*)	109	129	10
Active external rotation (*degrees*)	41	50	9
Active internal rotation (*10 points*)	5	7	2
Strength (*20 points*)	6	13	7
At 90° of flexion absolute Constant score (*100 points*)	44	77	33
Group 2: clavicular head of PM, *n* = 8 cases			
Pain (*15 points*)	0	13	13
Daily activities (*20 points*)	6	13	7
Active flexion (*degrees*)	168	163	-5
Active external rotation (*degrees*)	31	36	5
Active internal rotation (*10 points*)	0	7	7
Strength (*20 points*)	1	6	7
At 90° of flexion absolute Constant score (*100 points*)	29	61	32

*The values are given as the average and the range.

In the two groups, group 1: sternal head (n = 8 cases) and group 2: clavicular head (n = 7 cases), there was a significant improvement in the mean absolute Constant score between the pre- and the postoperative evaluations. So, the preoperative Constant score was different between the two groups but the gain did not differ significantly (Table II).

In this entire series, there was no significant correlation between the results of pectoralis major tendon transfer if the shoulder had previously operated or if the tendon transfer was the first operation. There was a correlation between the final result and the status of the supraspinatus (SS): the absolute constant score was higher when the supraspinatus was not torn or if the GFDI was less than 1 for supraspinatus and less than 2 for infraspinatus. But the gain of pectoralis major transfer was higher for a combined lesion of SS and subscapularis (Subscap) (anterosuperior lesion) (Table III).

Of the 15 patients who had had a positive lift off test preoperatively, 11 had a negative lift off test postoperatively. None of the two patients with a recurrent anterior instability preoperatively had a redislocation of the shoulder. One patient with a feeling of instability preoperatively had lost any sensation of anterior translation of the humeral head.

Of the 15 patients who had had a positive lift off test preoperatively, 11 had a negative lift off test postoperatively. Nine patients were manual workers and six were able to perform their work at the same level as before. The others patients who were retired or sedentary had returned to their earlier activities. Two MRI and one ultrasonography were performed at the latest follow-up. The flap was found to be well positioned, under the conjoined tendon and showed good trophicity of the muscle.

Table III – Final clinical results of PM transfer for combined SS and subscap lesion and isolated SS lesion*

	SS + Subscap			***Subscap isolated***		
	Pre-op	***Post-op***	***Gain***	***Pre-op***	***Post-op***	***Gain***
Pain (15 points)	3	13	10	7	15	8
Daily activities (*20 points*)	7	12	5	13	15	2
Active flexion (*degrees*)	149	145	-5	163	170	7
Active external rotation (*degrees*)	35	40	5	43	52	9
Active internal rotation (*10 points*)	2	7	5	7	9	2
Strength (*20 points*)	1			6		7
Absolute Constant score (*100 points*)	37	63	25	61	80	19

*The values are given as the average.

Complications

There were two postoperative complications, including one infection and one anterior chronic dislocation. The patient with a hematoma developed an infection with a rupture of the transferred pectoralis major. The patient was treated with an open debridement and an oral antibiotic for 6 weeks. The shoulder was pseudoparalytic with an absolute constant score of 41 points. The patient was disappointed and refused any revision. The second patient was a woman, 60 years old, with an anterosuperior degenerative lesion: MRI showed a fatty degeneration of the infraspinatus stage 3, a teres minor stage 2 (12), and an irreparable subscapularis tear retracted at the level of the glenoid with an atrophic muscle. The absolute constant score was 30 points. Pectoralis major tendon transfer alone was not able to restore active forward elevation and active external rotation. The humeral head escaped underneath the coraco-acromial arch and the shoulder was pseudoparalytic. A reverse prosthesis 6 months later was performed with a restoration of the active forward elevation and a patient satisfied at the latest follow-up.

Discussion

Transfer of the pectoralis major for the treatment of irreparable subscapularis tear has been already reported (10, 24-26), but different part of the pectoralis major and different ways to the lesser tuberosity have been described in the literature.

Young and Rockwood (27) were the first to use pectoralis major flap to treat a failure of Bristow technique for chronic anterior instability of the glenohumeral joint. The function of the pectoralis major (one case) was to reinforce a weak subscapularis muscle.

Wirth and Rockwood (10) reported a series of 16 patients with a chronic rupture of the subscapularis associated with a recurrent anterior instability of the shoulder. The superior half of the pectoralis major tendon was released from its insertion on the humerus in seven cases and passed over the conjoined tendon to be pull down to the bone trough at the level of the lesser tuberosity. The authors concluded that the pectoralis major muscle transferred was able to diminish anterior glenohumeral translation with the arm in external rotation.

Resch et al. (14) harvested the superior one half to two-thirds of the pectoralis major tendon from the humerus (which involves parts of both the sternal and the clavicular heads of the muscle), and reported a series of 12 patients with a mean postoperative absolute Constant score of 54.4 points (range 33-81 points). To reproduce the direction of the subscapularis muscle, the pectoralis major transfer was rerouted under the conjoined tendon.

Warner (23) used the sternal portion of the pectoralis major and preserved the clavicular portion. The sternal portion was rerouted underneath the clavicular portion and over the conjoined tendon to be fixed into the lesser tuberosity. He used the split pectoralis major transfer for 10 patients who were previously operated: failure of cuff repair (5 cases), failure of instability (3 cases), and 2 instability after hemiarthroplasty. All the patients recovered a stable shoulder with a pain relief but the functional gain was limited. No patient had a negative lift off test.

Vidil and Augereau (28) reported five patients with an irreparable subscapularis tear treated with a clavicular head of the pectoralis major moved over the horizontal part of the coracoid process. Four patients were followed up with an average absolute Constant score of 50 (range 30-63).

Jost et al. (13) released completely the pectoralis major tendon from its humeral insertion and transferred it to the less tuberosity over the conjoined tendon. Thirty pectoralis major transfer were performed for irreparable subscapularis tear isolated or associated with a rupture of the supraspinatus. There was a significant improvement in the scores for pain, activities of daily living, mobility, and abduction strength with a postoperative absolute average constant score of 62 points. Lift-off test remained positive in 23 of the 30 shoulders. Results are better if there is no concomitant rupture of the supraspinatus and/ or infraspinatus.

In the present clinical series, 13 shoulders were significantly improved, in terms of pain relief, activities of daily living, active range of motion, and strength, after a split pectoralis major transfer. Whatever the portion of the pectoralis major (clavicular or sternal), but always rerouted underneath the conjoined tendon, the results were comparable in those reported by Resch et al. (14) and Jost et al. (13). We did not find in this present clinical series any significant difference if we used the sternal or the clavicular portion of the pectoralis major to replace the function of the subscapularis.

Chaffai and Mansat (29) described the surgical anatomy of the pectoralis major and the possibility to transfer the clavicular portion for the reconstruction of an irreparable subscapularis tear. Neurovascular bundle was identified and recommendations for a safe surgery were already established.

To know which is the best portion of the pectoralis major is useful to harvest to reproduce the action of the subscapularis, Jennings et al. (30) dissected 22 fresh cadavers. They proved firstly the possibility to divide the sternal portion from the clavicular portion of the pectoralis major. Secondly, from a biomechanical standpoint they proved that the sternal portion rerouted underneath the clavicular portion and the conjoined tendon provide a transfer with a vector more closely matching that of the functioning subscapularis muscle. The authors concluded that the clavicular portion is biomechanically less efficient in providing the inferior vector than the sternal portion. The sternal portion of the pectoralis major can be transferred alone and create the best vector needed for the stabilization of the shoulder and to counteract the action of the deltoid.

Konrad et al. (31) compared the effects of the positioning of the PM tendon transfer above or underneath the conjoined tendon on the shoulder kinematics for subscapularis deficiency. From a biomechanical standpoint, they proved that the PM tendon transfer underneath the conjoined tendon reproduces closely the line of action of the subscapularis muscle. So they recommended to perform a pectoralis major tendon transfer underneath the conjoint tendon in subscapularis-deficient shoulders.

Combined tendon transfer has been proposed in global anteroposterior tear or in complete retracted subscapularis tear for young patient without arthritis. Galatz et al. (32) in anterosuperior and posterosuperior cuff tear with a pseudoparesis shoulder reported that the benefit of pectoralis major transfer anteriorly and latissimus dorsi transfer posteriorly was very limited. No pain but a mean active anterior elevation of 80° in 14 patients with a mean FU of 17.5 months.

Gerber et al. (33) proposed to do a double tendon transfer in patients with a complete rupture of the subscapularis. They transferred through an extended delto-pectoral approach the teres major to the inferior part of the lesser tuberosity and the sternal portion of the PM to the superior part of the lesser tuberosity. There was no significant difference in terms of pain, mobility, and strength between single or double transfer in 11 and 9 patients but they recommended double tendon transfer in patients with low and upper irreparable rupture of the subscapularis.

The pectoralis major transfer under the coracoid process in irreparable subscapularis tendon tear reduced the pain and improved the strength significantly. We did not find any difference in this short series if we used the clavicular head or the sternal head of the pectoralis major in spite of anatomical and biomechanical studies. Even though function is not completely restored in most patients, with lift off test and belly press test frequently positive postoperatively, a majority of patients recover an excellent shoulder function. Supraspinatus and infraspinatus degenerative lesion represents a negative prognosis factor for the final result of pectoralis major transfer.

References

1. Codman EA (1934) The shoulder. Rupture of the supraspinatus tendon and other lesions in or about the subacromial bursa. Boston: Privately printed; 262-312
2. Deutsch A, Altchek DW, Veltri DM, Potter HG, Warren RF (1997) Traumatic tears of the subscapularis tendon. Clinical diagnosis, magnetic resonance imaging findings, and operative treatment. Am J Sports Med; 25: 13-22
3. Frankle M, Cofield R (1992) Rotator cuff tears involving the subscapularis tendon. Techniques and results of repair. Read at the Fifth International Conference on Shoulder Surgery; July 12-15; Paris, France

4. Gerber C, Krushell RJ (1991) Isolated rupture of the tendon of the subscapularis muscle. Clinical features in 16 cases. J Bone Joint Surg Br; 73: 389-394
5. Nove-Josserand L, Gerber C, Walch G (1997) Lesions of the anterosuperior rotator cuff. In: Warner JPJ, Iannotti JP, Gerber C, editors. Complex and revision problems in shoulder surgery. Philadelphia: Lippincott-Raven; 165-176
6. Gerber C, Fuchs B, Hodler J (2000) The results of repair of massive tears of the rotator cuff. J Bone Joint Surg Am; 82: 505-515
7. Warner JJ, Higgins L, Parsons IM 4th, Dowdy P (2001) Diagnosis and treatment of anterosuperior rotator cuff tears. J Shoulder Elbow Surg; 10: 37-46
8. Hauser EDW (1954) Avulsion of the tendon of the subscapularis muscle. J Bone Joint Surg Am; 36: 139-141
9. Neviaser RJ, Neviaser TJ, Neviaser JS (1988) Concurrent rupture of the rotator cuff and anterior dislocation of the shoulder in the older patient. J Bone Joint Surg Am; 70: 1308-1311
10. Wirth MA, Rockwood CA Jr (1997) Operative treatment of irreparable rupture of the subscapularis. J Bone Joint Surg Am; 79: 722-731
11. Gerber C, Krushell RJ (1991) Isolated rupture of the tendon of the subscapularis muscle. Clinical features in 16 cases. J Bone Joint Surg Br; 73: 389-394
12. Goutallier D, Postel JM, Bernageau J, Lavau L, Voisin MC (1994) Fatty muscle degeneration in cuff ruptures. Pre- and postoperative evaluation by CT scan. Clin Orthop; 304: 78-83
13. Jost B, Puskas GJ, Lustenberger A, Gerber C (2003) Outcome of pectoralis major transfer for the treatment of irreparable subscapularis tears. J Bone Joint Surg Am; 85: 1944-1951
14. Resch H, Povacz P, Ritter E, Matschi W (2000) Transfer of the pectoralis major muscle for the treatment of irreparable rupture of the subscapularis tendon. J Bone Joint Surg Am; 82: 372-382
15. Constant CR, Murley AH (1987) A clinical method of functional assessment of the shoulder. Clin Orthop; 214: 160-164
16. Gerber C, Hersche O, Farron A (1996) Isolated rupture of the subscapularis tendon. J Bone Joint Surg Am; 78: 1015-1023
17. Gerber C, Nyffeler RW (2002) Classification of glenohumeral joint instability. Clin Orthop Relat Res; 400: 65-76
18. Nove-Josserand L, Levigne C, Noel E, Walch G (1994) Isolated lesions of the subscapularis muscle. Apropos of 21 cases. Rev Chir Orthop Reparatrice Appar Mot; 80: 595-601 (French)
19. Fuchs B, Weishaupt D, Zanetti M, Hodler J, Gerber C (1999) Fatty degeneration of the muscles of the rotator cuff: assessment by computed tomography versus magnetic resonance imaging. J Shoulder Elbow Surg; 8: 599-605
20. Samilson RL, Prieto V (1983) Dislocation arthropathy of the shoulder. J Bone Joint Surg Am; 65: 456-460

21. Klepps SJ, Goldfarb C, Flatow E, Galatz LM, Yamaguchi K (2001) Anatomic evaluation of the subcoracoid pectoralis major transfer in human cadavers. J Shoulder Elbow Surg; 10: 453-459
22. Elhassan B, Ozbaydar M, Massimini D, Diller D, Higgins L, Warner JJ (2008) Transfer of pectoralis major for the treatment of irreparable tears of subscapularis: does it work? J Bone Joint Surg Br; 90: 1059-1065
23. Warner JJ (2001) Management of massive irreparable rotator cuff tears: the role of tendon transfer. Instr Course Lect; 50: 63-71
24. Cofield RH, Parvizi J, Hoffmeyer PJ, Lanzer WL, Ilstrup DM, Rowland CM (2001) Surgical repair of chronic rotator cuff tears. A prospective long-term study. J Bone Joint Surg Am; 83: 71-77
25. Resch H, Povacz P, Ritter E, Matschi W (2000) Transfer of the pectoralis major muscle for the treatment of irreparable rupture of the subscapularis tendon. J Bone Joint Surg Am; 82: 372-382
26. Warner JJ (2001) Management of massive irreparable rotator cuff tears: the role of tendon transfer. Instr Course Lect; 50: 63-71
27. Young DC, Rockwood CA Jr (1991) Complications of a failed Bristow procedure and their management. J Bone Joint Surg Am; 73: 969-981
28. Vidil A, Augereau B (2000) Transfer of the clavicular portion of the pectoralis major muscle in the treatment of irreparable tears of the subscapularis muscle. Rev Chir Orthop Reparatrice Appar Mot; 86: 835-843 (French)
29. Chaffai MA, Mansat M (1988) Anatomic bases for the reconstruction of a musculotendinous flap derived from the pectoralis major muscle. Surg Radiol Anat; 10: 273-282
30. Jennings GJ, Keereweer S, Buijze GA, De Beer J, DuToit D (2007) Transfer of segmentally split pectoralis major for the treatment of irreparable rupture of the subscapularis tendon. J Shoulder Elbow Surg; 16: 837-842
31. Konrad GG, Sudkamp NP, Kreuz PC, Jolly JT, McMahon PJ, Debski RE (2007) Pectoralis major tendon transfers above or underneath the conjoint tendon in subscapularis-deficient shoulders. An in vitro biomechanical analysis. J Bone Joint Surg Am; 89: 2477-2484
32. Galatz LM, Connor PM, Calfee RP, Hsu JC, Yamaguchi K (2003) Pectoralis major transfer for anterior-superior subluxation in massive rotator cuff insufficiency. J Shoulder Elbow Surg; 12: 1-5
33. Gerbert C, Clavert P, Millet PJ, Holovacs TF, Warner JJP (2004) Split pectoralis major and teres major tendon transfers for reconstruction of irreparable tears of the subscapularis. Tech Shoulder Elbow Surg; 5: 5-12

Reverse shoulder prosthesis combined with latissimus dorsi and teres major transfer for a lack of active elevation and external rotation

Ph. Valenti, A. Kilinc, L. Thomsen

Historical perspective: Introduction

In massive irreparable cuff tear, loss of active elevation and external rotation of the shoulder is very rare. The lack of active external rotation with the arm at the side (ER1) or in 90° of abduction (ER2) is associated with a severe atrophy or fatty infiltration of the infraspinatus (IS) and teres minor (Tm) (1, 2).

External rotation is useful for daily activities and particularly to bring hand to the mouth, to eat, to drink, to brush teeth, or to work with the arm overhead such as combing hair. Loss of active external rotation with the arm at the side is documented by a dropping sign and an external lag sign. If the patient can elevate upper limb at the horizontal level, an hornblower sign appears when the patient tries to reach his/her mouth (3, 4).

In elderly patients, with a pseudoparalytic shoulder secondary to rotator cuff deficiency, reverse shoulder prosthesis (RSP) has proved to be the gold standard to restore an active forward flexion or abduction (5-7). But active external rotation is not improved after RSP and clinical outcome is poorer in the absence of residual Tm (8). Less medialized RSP has reported better external rotation than original delta prosthesis but a good trophicity of the Tm is needed (9, 10).

In Erb's palsy, for pediatric population, L'Episcopo in 1934 described a rerouted of teres major (TM) around the humerus to restore active external rotation with a posterior and anterior approach (11). Later, Zachary noted that "latissimus dorsi (LD) was so intimely blended with TM" and could be taken both (12). Merle d'Aubigne and Gerard in 1947 reported a rerouted of LD and TM around the humerus, with a single approach: deltopectoral or axillary.

The two tendons transplanted were sutured to the pectoralis major (PM) with arm in external rotation (13).

Wickstrom et al., Hoffer et al., and Gilbert and Tassin reported in obstetrical brachial palsy with a lack of external rotation, excellent results of LD transfer to the supraspinatus (SS) insertion regarding recovery of forward elevation and external rotation (12, 14-16). Gerber et al. thought that massive cuff tear in adult constituted a similar problem and reported the first 14 cases of LD transfer fixed to the bone at the level of the insertion of SS; they reported a gain both external rotation and forward flexion (17).

Based on this both experience, Gerber et al. in 2007 reported a preliminary report of 12 cases of combination of LD transfer to the great tuberosity with an RSP for patients with a loss of active external rotation (18). He concluded with a small number of patients and a relatively short follow-up (FU) a significant improvement of the score of functional active external rotation (4.6-8.2 of 10 points) and daily living (2.3-7.9 of 10 points) but with a non-significant improvement of active external rotation with the arm at the side (from 12° to 19°).

Boileau et al. in 2007 reported six cases of combination of LD and TM transfer on the posterolateral aspect of the greater tuberosity (at the infraspinatus and Tm insertion) (19). The mean increase of active external rotation was 28.3° and 30 points of gain according to Constant score (20).

We report our experience regarding five patients with an active anterior elevation less 60° with less 0° of active external rotation the arm at the side in neutral position secondary to an irreparable posterosuperior cuff tear with a Tm atrophic with a fatty infiltration >3. Our procedure combined an RSP and LD and TM transfer fixed on the lateral aspect of the humerus at the level of their insertion.

Indications and contraindications

Patient with a chronic pseudoparesis shoulder (<60°active forward flexion) and a dynamic superior and anterior migration of the humeral head (after 6 months of physiotherapy) when he/she tries to elevate the arm is candidate to RSP. With a loss of external rotation the arm at the side or in abduction less than 60° is candidate to RSP combined with LD and TM tendon transfer to restore active external rotation. These situations may be the result of failed hemiarthroplasty or sequelae of complex fracture with a migration or osteolysis of the great tuberosity, a failed repair of massive posterosuperior cuff tear or after an acromioplasty in irreparable anterosuperior tear. We extended our indications for patient with an hornblower' sign and eccentric arthritis of the glenohumeral joint (stage 3-4 in Hamada classification) (21).

Palsy of the deltoid, previous infection, or glenoid bone deficiency (bone loss or osteoporotic that cannot authorized implantation of a semi-constrained prosthesis) are contraindications of RSP.

A relative contraindication is the young patient without arthritis (stage 1-2 in Hamada classification) and an anterior and posterior irreparable cuff tear; Aldridge et al. in young patients tried to make a combination of tendon transfer (22). He reported a retrospective review of 11 consecutive patients treated with a combined transfer of the LD and PM tendons for massive rotator cuff deficiency involving both anterior and posterior cuff. Only 50% of the patients were improved with a gain of 44° in elevation and 13° in external rotation. These authors recommended this salvage procedure only for young patients under 60 years old with a massive tear involving the anterior and posterior cuff in which the coraco-acromial (CA) ligament is not torn.

Preoperative planning

Clinical evaluation was performed in all patients before operation and at the postoperative FU, using the 100-point rating system of Constant (pain on a scale of 15 points, activity of daily living 20 points, and strength 25 points) (20). Range of active and passive movement were recorded for forward elevation and abduction, external rotation with the arm at the side (ER1), external rotation in 90° of abduction (ER2), and for internal rotation.

Clinical examination confirmed functional signs of loss active forward elevation and external rotation: patients were unable to reach 90° of anterior elevation and with the arm at the side, active external rotation was less 0°. Severe deficiency of active external rotation was documented by positive external lag sign or a dropping sign. A hornblower' sign appeared when the patient tried to reach the mouth with his/her hand (4, 23).

Pre- and postoperative radiographs included anteroposterior (AP), outlet, and axillary views: AP view defined the acromio-humeral space; outlet view (static and dynamic) appreciated the superior and anterior migration of the humeral head under the CA arch. Axillary view measured the size of the glenoid, degree of retroversion, and the quantity of bone to implant a metaglene. Post-op radiographs looked for radiolucents lines and glenoid notch according Nérot'radiological classification and metaphysic osteolysis (24).

Magnetic resonance imaging showed the degree of atrophy and fatty infiltration of SS, IS, and Tm according to the system of Thomazeau et al. and Goutallier et al., a superior or posterosuperior abrasion of the glenoid (2, 25, 26).

Techniques

Surgical approach (Figs. 1 and 2)

The patient is placed in "semi-sitting" beach chair position with the entire upper limb draped in the operative field. The arm should be free to facilitate expositioning of the glenoid and harvesting and securing the transferred tendons. We use a standard deltopectoral approach extended distally to the deltoid insertion on the humerus. Incision begins from the clavicle to the inferior border of the PM tendon, following the deltopectoral interval outside the coracoid. The cephalic vein is retracted laterally. Axillary and musculocutaneous nerves should be identified with the index finger before inserting the retractor under the conjoint tendon and the anterior fibers of the deltoid. The irreparable character of the massive rupture of SS and IS is confirmed with the arm in retropulsion, abduction, and medial rotation. If the long head of the biceps is still present, it is always pathologic in this context. Then, we perform a tenodesis in the superior part of the bicipital groove with local soft tissue with an absorbable suture (Vicryl No. 2-0; Ethicon®); intra-articular portion is resected. Frequently, the superior part of the subscapularis is frayed or partially torn. With the arm in external rotation and forward flexion we ligate the anterior circonflex vessels before cutting the subscapularis at the myotendinous junction. We cut the capsule at the same level and we left a lateral stump of subscapularis to reattach it at the end of the operation. We release, the coraco-humeral ligament and the superior border of the subscapularis under the coracoid process in order to obtain a better gliding of the subscapularis tendon.

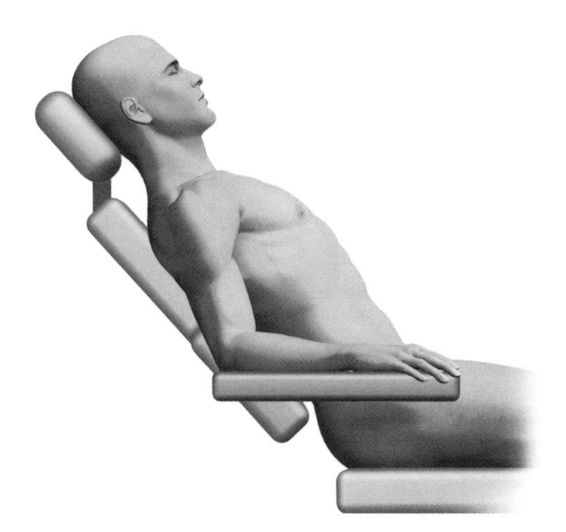

Fig. 1 – Semi sitting"Beach chair position.

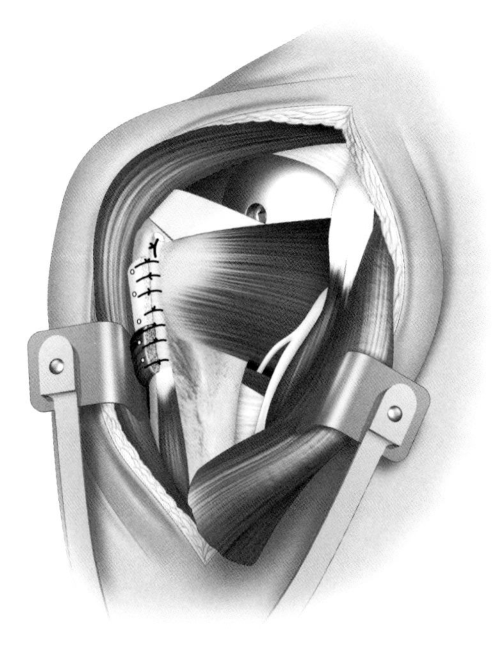

Fig. 2 – Extended delto pectoral approach
D: Deltoid muscle; B: Long Biceps; CT: Conjoint tendon; SS: Subscapularis; PM: Pectoralis major; TM: Teres major; LD: Latissimus dorsi.

Harvesting and preparation of rerouted LD and TM transfer (Figs. 3 and 4)

We first identify the long head of the biceps, at the inferior part of the incision, which runs vertically and posteriorly to the tendinous insertion of PM. We protect with scissor the biceps tendon and we cut the upper half of the PM 1 cm medial to the humeral insertion. We leave a lateral stump of the PM to reattach it and to suture to the transferred LD tendon. The medial stump of PM is retracted medially with stay sutures allowing a good exposition of the tendinous portion of the LD and TM. The LD is always located anteriorly to the TM tendon (slightly inferiorly) at the humeral insertion site. Sometimes their insertion seems to form a conjoint unit that we can separate with a sharp dissection. The average length of the tendinous portion of LD (8.4 cm: 6.3-10.1) is longer than TM (3.9 cm: 3.3-4.6) and facilitate to pass stay sutures and to fix it on the lateral aspect of the humerus (24). Before cutting and releasing the two tendons, it is important to remember anatomical position of the axillary and radial nerve and neurovascular bundles of these two tendons (25). The distance between the insertion of these two tendons on the medial aspect of the humerus and the nerves depends on the position of the arm:

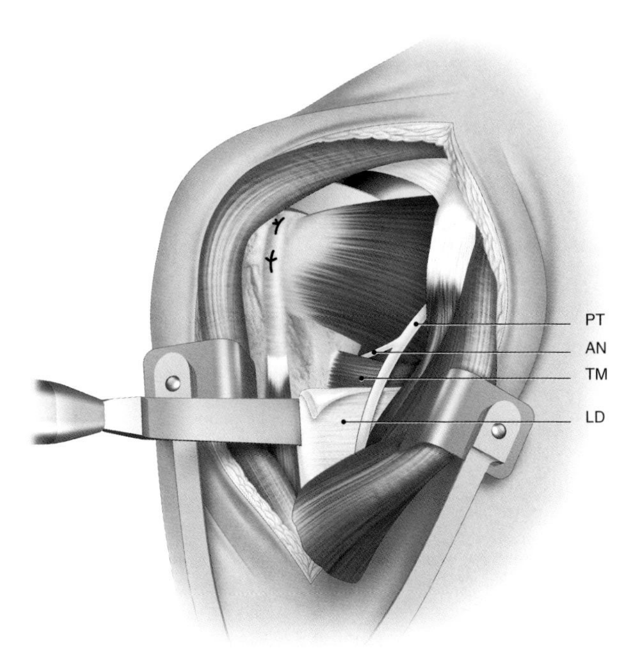

Fig. 3 – Latissimus dorsi anteriorly and teres major posteriorly are isolated from the humerus. PT: Posterior cord; AN: Axillary nerve; TM: Teres major; LD: Latissimus dorsi.

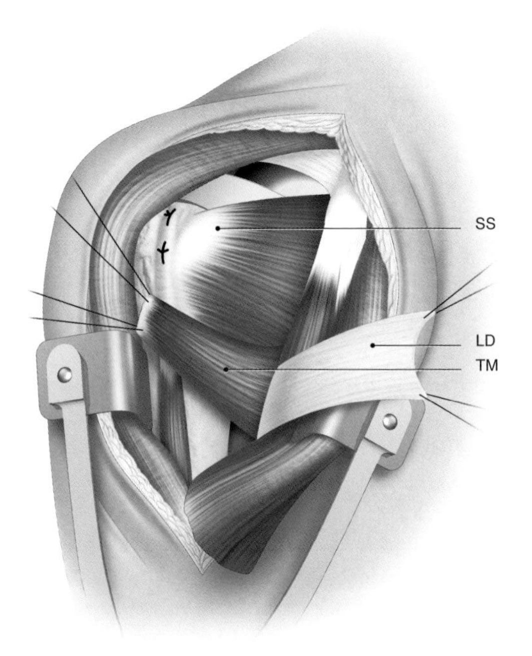

Fig. 4 – Release medially LD and TM be careful to radial nerve and axillary nerve. SS: Subscapularis; TM: Teres major; LD: Latissimus dorsi.

with an anterior approach, the distance decreases in abduction and external rotation and increases in adduction and neutral rotation. Axillary nerve after travelling along the anteroinferior border of the subscapularis muscle crossed horizontally the quadrilateral space bounded by Tm superiorly, long head of triceps medially, superior border of TM, and surgical neck of the humerus laterally. The axillary nerve is divided into a posterior trunk to innervate Tm and posterior fibers of the deltoid, and anterior trunk to supply medial and anterior fibers of the deltoid. The radial nerve runs vertically over the anterior surface of the two tendons. With the arm in adduction and neutral rotation, radial nerve is located at an average of 2.9 cm (range 2.0-4.0 cm) medial to the surgical neck of the humerus (27). Distal to the tendons, radial nerve arrives in the posterior compartment to the bone spiral groove.

The release of the two tendons medially should be safe to avoid neurovascular bundles lesion and particularly for the TM: the lower subscapular nerve enters the anterior aspect of the TM muscle at an average of 7.4 cm (±1.4) medial to its humeral insertion; the thoraco-dorsal nerve enters the LD at an average of 13.1 cm (±1.8) medial to its humeral insertion.

We detach with the scalpel LD and TM from the humerus with periosteal tissue to reinforce the tendinous portion. Stay non-absorbable sutures (ethibond no. 3; Ethicon) are placed into the two tendinous stumps with some difficulties in TM, which is more muscular. A gentle atraumatic medially release allows to individualize LD and TM. The potential excursion of 33.9 cm of LD compared to 14.9 cm of TM explains the facilities to pull around the humerus of LD. So, as we know after the study of Herzberg and with the inconvenient of a small tendinous portion for the TM, the combined tendon transfer (LD and TM) bring a strength closed to IS and Tm and has been recommended Mansat and co-workers (28, 29).

When both the tendons are fully mobilized, a curved clamp is guided around the surgical neck of the humerus, close to the bone, at the level of their insertion creating a tunnel for tendon passage. The stay sutures of the two tendons are grasped with a clamp and left on the lateral aspect of the humerus to be secured after implantation and reduction of the RSP (Figs. 5 and 5bis).

Preparation of the humerus

The bone cut of the humeral head begins at the junction of the cephalic cartilage and greater tuberosity with an inclination of 155° and an average retroversion of 20°. This cut should be ended at the inferior border of the glenoid to facilitate reduction of the prosthesis. Metaphysis and epiphysis are prepared with progressive larger graspers. The goal is to retain as much cancellous bone in the metaphysis part as possible providing a press fit fixation for the humeral stem. To obtain an excellent primary stability we impact cancellous bone graft (from the humeral head) in the medial part of the metaphysis. We prefer cementless humeral stem but we use cement into the diaphysis for elderly

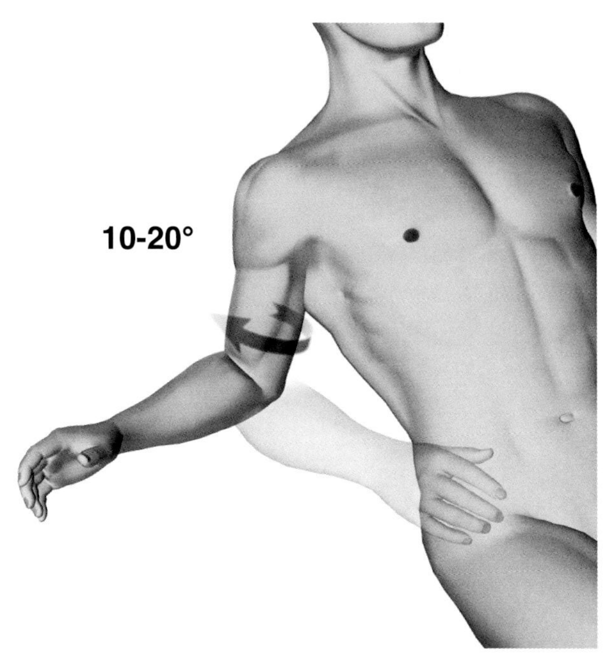

Fig. 5 – Episcopo procedure with the upper limb In external rotation.

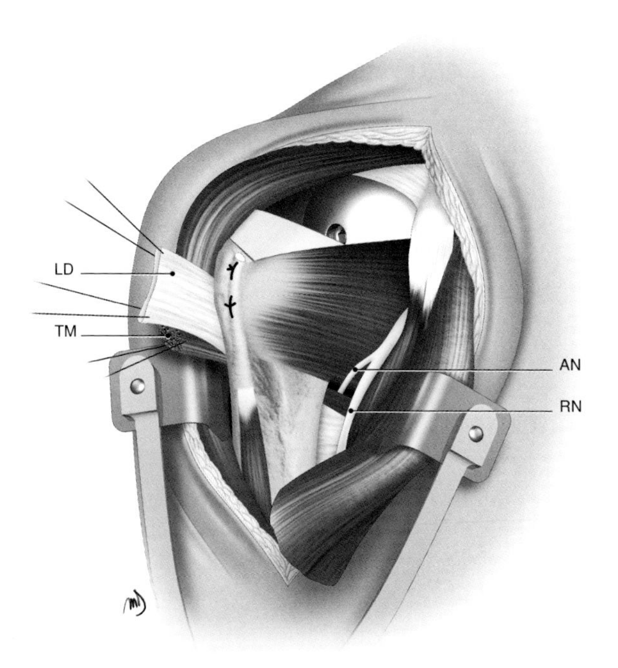

Fig.5bis – LD and TM are rerouted around the humerus and fixed to the lateral aspect of the great tuberosity.
RN: Radial nerve; AN: Axillary nerve; TM: Teres major; LD: Latissimus dorsi.

patients with osteoporotic bone and if the trial component moves into the metaphysis. The design of this universal stem creates a lateralization of 3 mm compared to the traditional shape of the delta prosthesis (Depuy®).

Preparation of the glenoid

The upper end of the humerus is retracted inferiorly and posteriorly with the arm in forward flexion to obtain a good exposition of the inferior part of the glenoid. The capsule is circumferentially excised from the glenoid, staying in contact with the glenoid bone to avoid axillary nerve damage. The anterior retractor gives the orientation of the glenoid and facilitates positioning of the central hole with the stopper drill. The articular cartilage is removed to the level of subchondral bone to medialize the glenosphere according Grammont's concepts. Great care should be necessary if the bone is fragile, osteoporotic, or in eccentric head with osteolysis of the acromion and no constraints over the glenoid. The metal back (MB) is positioned as low as possible in a plane perpendicular to the glenoid. A superior tilt (caused by a bad exposition) is a technical fault and explains the risk of early glenoid loosening. A superior or a postero-superior glenoid abrasion should be grafted to avoid malposition of the MB. The back shape of the MB is convex, with a central keel and an anterior plate covered with hydroxyl apatite, providing an excellent press fit fixation to counter shearing forces at the MB-bone interface in the first degrees of the abduction. Two divergent screws provide definitive fixing of this MB. This excellent quality of fixation authorized us to use a glenosphere applied over the MB and not embedded to create a lateralization of the center of rotation (8.7 mm).

Reduction of the prosthesis

The trial humeral cup is impacted into the definitive humeral stem and the joint is reduced by lowering and abducting the arm, allowing the humeral cup to slide under the glenosphere. The polyethylene cup of the Arrow RSP is deeper than the traditional delta with a better primary stability and we recommend not to make the joint too tight. Our experience suggests that between 0° and 60° of abduction in the glenohumeral joint, we create any movement of the scapula. Scapular tilting within a few degrees of abduction suggests that the prosthesis is too tight, and a more extensive soft tissue release or further humeral metaphysis bone has to be performed. If the prosthesis seems too unstable it is possible to use a thicker humeral stem (+5, +10 mm) or a larger sized glenosphere (size 39). Any impingement should be created with a gap between glenosphere and PE cup in adduction (osteophyte glenoid pillar) or abduction (acromion) or in medial rotation (coracoids), or in external rotation (posterior glenoid).

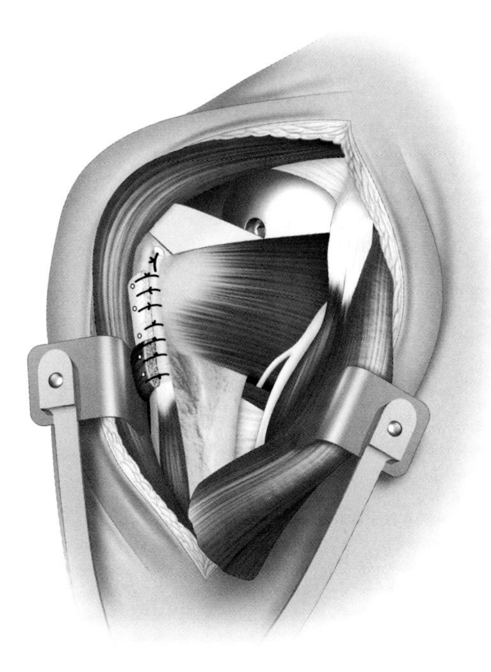

Fig. 6 – LD and TM fixed on the lateral aspect of the great tuberosity. Tenodesis of the Long head of bicepsAnd repair of the subscapularis.

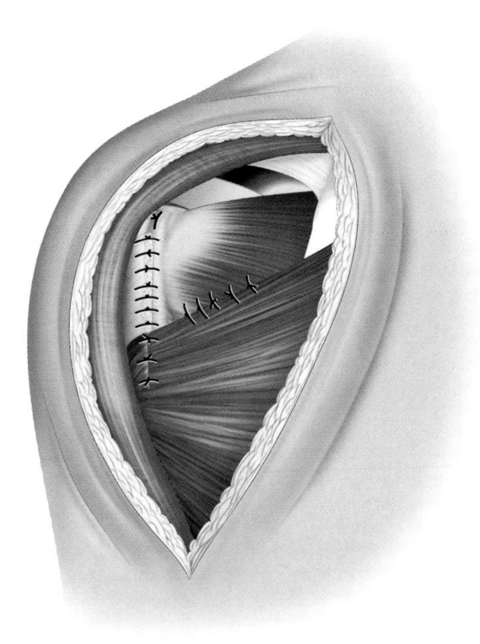

Fig. 7 – Finally repair of the pectoralis major.

Fixation of the both transferred tendons (Figs. 6 and 7)

The arm is positioned in abduction 30° and external rotation of approximately 60°. The two stay sutures of the LD tendon were fixed transosseously with two bone anchors (Super G4 Mitek; Depuy) closed to the distal part of the bicipital groove. The two stay sutures of TM tendon are fixed more laterally (less potential of excursion, short and bulky muscle) with two others bone anchors. To reinforce their fixation we suture both LD and TM with the lateral and medial stumps of PM and the biceps tendon. The subscapularis is reattached transosseously in the medial aspect of the less tuberosity (lateralization of the humerus with Arrow RSP). The deltopectoral incision is also closed over one drain for 48 h, and the arm is placed in 20° of abduction and in 30° of external rotation in a special brace.

Postoperative management

The brace in 20° of abduction and 30° of external rotation is applied for 6 weeks. Mobilization of the hand and the elbow with passive pendulum exercises are encouraged immediately after the operation. Passive ROM in elevation and external rotation until neutral rotation is authorized after 6 weeks. Balneotherapy and internal rotation is allowed after 12 weeks with a physiotherapy program of reinforcement of lowering and external muscles for 3-6 months.

Results and complications

We excluded four patients: three with a lack of external rotation and a complete forward elevation who were treated by an Episcopo procedure without RSP and another with an osteoarthritis of the glenohumeral joint and an atrophy of IS and Tm had been treated with an anatomic total shoulder arthroplasty and LD and TM transfer.

Five patients (two women and three men; average age 68.8 years) with a combined pseudoparesis of forward elevation with a lack of external rotation were treated by an RSP and LD and TM transfer according to Episcopo procedure. All the patients had been reviewed with a minimal of 12 months of FU and an average of 26.4 months (range 12-48 months). One patient had a transient high radial palsy with a complete recovery in 3 months. The absolute Constant's score improved from 24.8 preoperatively to 57.20 at the latest FU: the gain in forward flexion was 74° (average 46° pre-op to 120° post-op) and in external rotation the arm at the side was 50° (–20° pre-op to 30° post-op). While improvement of external rotation is highly significant, medial rotation did not decrease significantly (5.6 pre-op to 5.2 post) of

10 points according to the system of Constant. All patients were satisfied or very satisfied at the last review and the score according to the simple shoulder test (refe) improved from 2 points preoperatively to 9 points postoperatively of 12 points. The worst result was a stiff shoulder secondary to a complex fracture treated by three previous operations (nail, hemiarthroplasty, and surgical arthrolysis). Pseudoparalytic shoulder with a complete passive range of motion (failure of repair massive cuff tear) represents the best candidate for this combined operation.

We have not seen any glenoid notching with this less medialized RSP (Arrow, FH, Mulhouse, France) and a normal aspect of the shoulder contour. We have not seen any instability, any infection, and any glenoid loosening in this series that addressed to the patients with a minimal of three previous operations.

Conclusion

We believe that this preliminary report of combined RSP and LD and TM transfer around the surgical neck of the humerus at the level of Tm represent a reliable technique to treat a loss of active anterior elevation and external rotation. This operation is such longer and more sophisticated than RSP alone but the rate of complication is not increased and the benefit for daily activities is evident. Biggest serie and longer FU and further studies should be necessary to validate definitively this procedure.

References

1. Fuchs B, Weishaupt D, Zanetti M, et al. (1999) Fatty degeneration of the muscles of the rotator cuff: assessment by computed tomography versus magnetic resonance imaging. J Shoulder Elbow Surg; 8: 599-605
2. Goutallier D, Postel JM, Bernageau J, et al. (1994) Fatty muscle degeneration in cuff ruptures. Pre- and postoperative evaluation by CT Scan. Clin Orthop Relat Res; 304: 78-83
3. Walch G, Boulahia A, Calderone S, et al. (1998) The dropping and hornblower's signs in evaluation of rotator cuff tears. J Bone Joint Surg Br; 80: 624-628
4. Hertel R, Ballmer FT, Lambert SM, et al. (1996) Lag signs in the diagnosis of rotator cuff rupture. J Shoulder Elbow Surg; 5: 307-313
5. Sirveaux F, Favard L, Oudet D, et al. (2004) Grammont inverted total shoulder arthroplasty in the treatment of glenohumeral osteoarthritis with massive rupture of the cuff. Results of a multicentre study of 80 shoulders. J Bone Joint Surg Br; 86: 388-395

6. Boileau P, Watkinson DJ, Hatzidakis AM, et al. (2005) Grammont reverse prosthesis: design, rationale, and biomechanics. J Shoulder Elbow Surg; 14: 147S-161S
7. Werner CM, Steinmann PA, Gilbart M, et al. (2005) Treatment of painful pseudoparesis due to irreparable rotator cuff dysfunction with the delta III reverse-ball-and-socket total shoulder prosthesis. J Bone Joint Surg Am; 87: 1476-1486
8. Simovitch RW, Helmy N, Zumstein MA, et al. (2007) Impact of fatty infiltration of the teres minor muscle on the outcome of reverse total shoulder arthroplasty. J Bone Joint Surg Am; 89: 934-939
9. Frankle M, Siegal S, Pupello D, et al. (2005) The reverse shoulder prosthesis for glenohumeral arthritis associated with severe rotator cuff deficiency. A minimum two-year follow-up study of sixty patients. J Bone Joint Surg Am; 87: 1697-1705
10. Baulot E, Chabernaud D, Grammont PM (1995) Results of grammont's inverted prosthesis in omarthritis associated with major cuff destruction. A propos of 16 cases. Acta Orthop Belg; 61: 112S-119S (in French)
11. L'Episcopo JB (1934) Tendon transplantation in obstetrical paralysis. Am J Surg; 25: 122-125
12. Zachary RB (1947) Transplantation of teres major and latissimus dorsi for loss of external rotation at shoulder. Lancet; 250: 757-758
13. Merle D'Aubigné R (1947) Paralysie du plexus brachial traitée par transposition des tendons grand rond et grand dorsal. Memoires De L'académie De Chirurgie
14. Wickstrom J, Haslam ET, Hutchinson Rh (1955) The surgical management of residual deformities of the shoulder following birth injuries of the brachial plexus. J Bone Joint Surg Am; 37: 27-36
15. Hoffer MM, Wickenden R, Roper B (1978) Brachial plexus birth palsies. Results of tendon transfers to the rotator cuff. J Bone Joint Surg Am; 60: 691-695
16. Gilbert A, Tassin JL (1984) Surgical repair of the brachial plexus in obstetric paralysis. Chirurgie; 110: 70-75 (in French)
17. Gerber C, Vinh TS, Hertel R, et al. (1988) Latissimus dorsi transfer for the treatment of massive tears of the rotator cuff. A preliminary report. Clin Orthop Relat Res; 232: 51-61
18. Gerber C, Pennington SD, Lingenfelter EJ, et al. (2007) Reverse delta-III total shoulder replacement combined with latissimus dorsi transfer. A preliminary report. J Bone Joint Surg Am; 89: 940-947
19. Boileau P, Trojani CH, Chuinard C (2007) Latissimus dorsi and teres major transfer with reverse total shoulder arthroplasty for a combined loss of elevation and external rotation. Tech in Shoulder Elbow Surg: 8; 13-22
20. Constant CR, Murley AH (1987) A clinical method of functional assessment of the shoulder. Clin Orthop Relat Res; 214: 160-164
21. Hamada K, Fukuda H, Mikasa M, et al. (1990) Roentgenographic findings in massive rotator cuff tears. A long-term observation. Clin Orthop Relat Res; 254: 92-96

22. Aldridge JM 3rd, Atkinson TS, Mallon WJ (2004) Combined pectoralis major and latissimus dorsi tendon transfer for massive rotator cuff deficiency. J Shoulder Elbow Surg; 13: 621-629
23. Walch G, Boulahia A, Calderone S, et al. (1998) The dropping and hornblower's signs in evaluation of rotator cuff tears. J Bone Joint Surg Br; 80: 624-628
24. Valenti PH, Boutens D, Nérot C (2001) Delta 3 reversed prosthesis for osteoarthritis with massive rotator cuff tear: long term results. In: Walch G, Boileau P, Molé D, editors. 2000 Prothèses D'épaule... Recul De 2 A 10 Ans. Paris: Sauramps Médical: 253-259 (in French)
25. McClelland D, Paxinos A (2008) The anatomy of the quadrilateral space with reference to quadrilateral space syndrome. J Shoulder Elbow Surg; 17: 162-164
26. Thomazeau H, Boukobza E, Morcet N, et al. (1997) Prediction of rotator cuff repair results by magnetic resonance imaging. Clin Orthop; 344: 275-283
27. Pearle AD, Voos JE, Kelly BT, et al. (2007) Surgical technique and anatomic study of latissimus dorsi and teres major transfers. J Bone Joint Surg Am; 89: 284-296
28. Herzberg G, Urien JP, Dimnet J (1999) Potential excursion and relative tension of muscles in the shoulder girdle relevance to tendon transfer. J Shoulder Elbow Surg; 8: 430-437
29. Combes JM, Mansat M (1995) Traitement des rutures massives de la colffe des rotateurs par lambeau du muscle gland rond. In: Bonnel F, editor. Ch Epaule Musculaire Montpelller: Sauramps Médical: 227-236

Algorithm of indications in symptomatic irreparable cuff tear

Ph. Valenti

Irreparable rotator cuff tear are rare and may present with a variety of clinical manifestations and distinct anatomic patterns. A rotator cuff tear is defined as irreparable if the quality of the tendon is so poor that direct tendon to bone repair is not possible and/or the muscle is atrophic or infiltrated stage III or IV regarding Goutallier classification. There are two distinct anatomic patterns: the posterosuperior tear involves the supraspinatus (SS) and the infraspinatus (IS) and the less common anterosuperior tear involves the subscapularis and the supraspinatus. The posterosuperior tear can be extended to the teres minor with a lack of active external rotation and a positive drop sign or hornblower sign. Very infrequently the posterosuperior tear can be extended anteriorly to the subscapularis defined as a "global" irreparable rotator cuff tear.

Indications and contraindications of tendon transfer in irreparable rotator cuff tear depend on general factors, clinical and imaging evaluation. So, many factors should be discussed as the age (young, older), degree of motivation of the patient, capacity to follow rehabilitation, degree of pain and weakness of the shoulder, status of the long head of the biceps, degree of lack of range of motion (active forward elevation, external rotation of the arm at the side and in 90° of abduction), drop sign, lack sign of external rotation, lift off test, belly press test, arthritis of glenohumeral joint, and status of the coraco-acromial arch (efficiency or not).

Tendon transfer is contraindicated for:

– older patients with a low demanding;
– patients with a good range of motion and no pain after physiotherapy;
– pseudoparalytic shoulder (AAE less 60°) with an escape of the humeral head anteriorly and superiorly underneath the coraco-acromial arch;
– deltoid palsy;
– glenohumeral arthritis (Samilson II or III) but tendon transfer can be combined with a reverse shoulder prosthesis (RSP) to restore active external rotation in patients with an atrophic teres minor.

Indications (Fig. 1)

Tendon transfer may be proposed in young patients who have both pain and weak shoulder, and/or a loss of active anterior elevation and/or a loss of active external rotation.

Two types of anatomic patterns can be managed:

A posterosuperior tear (involves SS and IS) can be repaired currently with a latissimus dorsi transfer or less frequently, in Europe with a deltoid flap. The location of the insertion of the LD transfer depends on degree of active external rotation; if there is an hornblower sign, we fix the LD on the insertion of the infraspinatus in over the great tuberosity; if the lack is in the sector of active anterior elevation, the LD will be fixed at the insertion of supraspinatus closed to the subscapularis. A teres major transfer is a reasonable choice for infraspinatus tear or posterosuperior tear with a loss of active external rotation.

An anterosuperior tear (involves SS and subscapularis) can be repaired with the pectoralis major. A split of the pectoralis major is the method of choice in chronic isolated subscapularis tear. When the subscapularis is completely torn with a lift off test positif, we combined the teres major in the lower portion of the lesser tuberosity and the pectoralis major in the superior portion of the lesser tuberosity. There is no significant difference clinically between sternal head and clavicular head rerouted underneath the conjoined tendon.

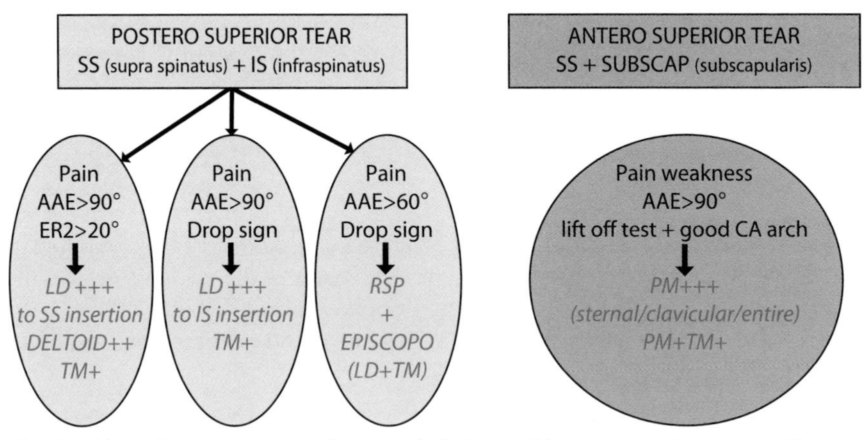

Fig. 1 – Algorythm treatment: tendon transfer in irreparable symptomatic rotator cuff tear. +++ first choice; ++ second choice; + third choice; AAE: active anterior; ER2: external rotation at 90° of abduction; LD: latissimus dorsi; TM: teres major; PM: pectoralis major; RSP: reverse shoulder prosthesis.

If the posterosuperior tear is associated with a glenohumeral arthritis, and a pseudoparalytic shoulder, the RSP is the method of choice to restore active forward elevation. RSP is not able to restore external rotation if there is an atrophic teres minor and we reroute latissimus dorsi and teres major around the humerus at the same level to fix them on the lateral aspect of the humerus (Episcopo procedure).

Algorythm treatment for tendon transfer in irreparable symptomatic rotator cuff tear (Fig. 2).

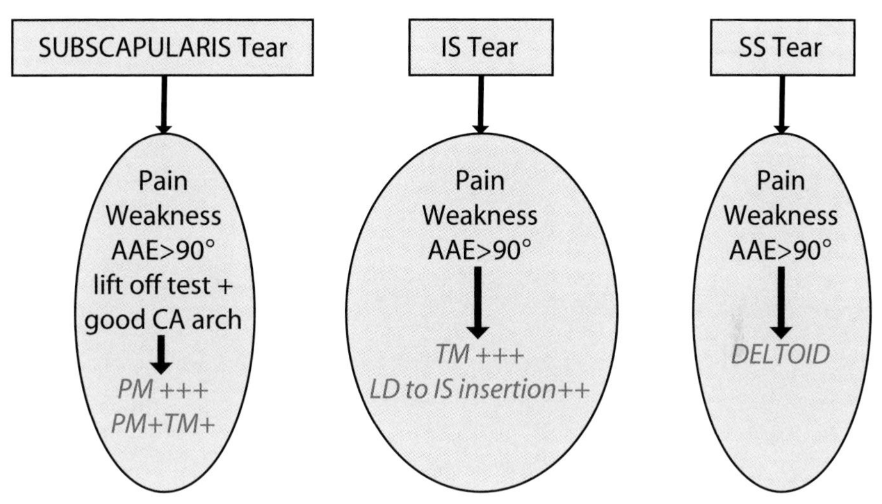

Fig. 2 – Algorythm treatment: tendon transfer in irreparable symptomatic rotator cuff tear. PM: pectoralis major; TM: teres major; AAE: active anterior elevation; IS: infra spinatus; SS:supraspinatus; LD: latissimus dorsi; CA: coraco acronimial.

Achevé d'imprimer par
l'Imprimerie Vasti-Dumas - 42010 Saint-Etienne
Dépôt légal : octobre 2010
N° d'imprimeur : V006069/00

Imprimé en France